Nothing
To Lose
But
The Pain

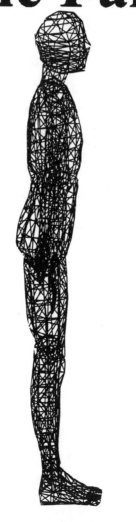

Patient was first seen in the office several years ago, having suffered chronic pain in various parts of her body since childhood and needing ongoing chiropractic and osteopathic care. She had chronic jaw, mid and low back pains. She had recurrent and long-lasting headaches. She had pain in her left foot and also developed a sciatica and a thoracic outlet syndrome problem on the right side.
After undergoing Posture Control Therapy, without any drugs or surgery, her symptoms receded.

Nothing To Lose But The Pain

Without Drugs or Surgery

For Relief of Postural Pains:
Foot To Jaw

By Dr. Myles J. Schneider

Foreword by Bernard E. Filner, M.D.

Published by
Acropolis South L.C.

NOTHING TO LOSE BUT THE PAIN by Myles J. Schneider

If unavailable in local bookstores, additional copies may be
purchased by writing to the Acropolis Customer Service Dept.,
415 Wood Duck Drive, Sarasota, FL 34236.
(Phone 813-953-5214/FAX 813-366-0745)

Printed in the United States of America.

LIBRARY OF CONGRESS CATALOGING-IN-PUBLICATION DATA

Schneider, Myles J.
    Nothing to lose but the pain , without drugs or surgery : for
relief of postural pains — foot to jaw / by Myles J. Schneider.
      p.   cm.
    Includes bibliographical references and index.
    ISBN 0-8749-1985-1
    1. Posture disorders. 2. Pain—Treatment. 3. Orthopedic shoes.
I. Title.
RD762.S35 1995
617.3–dc20   95-18101
                                        CIP

Other Books by Myles J. Schneider:

The Family Foot Care Book with Mark D. Sussman (Acropolis)
How to Doctor Your Feet Without A Doctor
   with Mark D. Sussman (Acropolis)
The Athlete's Healthcare Book with Mark D. Sussman (Acropolis)
Divorce Mediation with Karen L. Schneider (Acropolis)

Dedication

To my best friend and beautiful wife "Shana" (Sharon) and our wonderful family: Frank, Sam, Charissa, David and Jessica. — *M J S*

Quiz

Do you . . .

☐   Suffer from pains in the neck, back, legs?

Have you . . .

☐   Had medical treatment with limited or unsatisfactory results?

☐   Had to alter your lifestyle? Occupation? Fitness activities? due to pain.

Do you . . .

☐   Want help?

Then this book is for you!

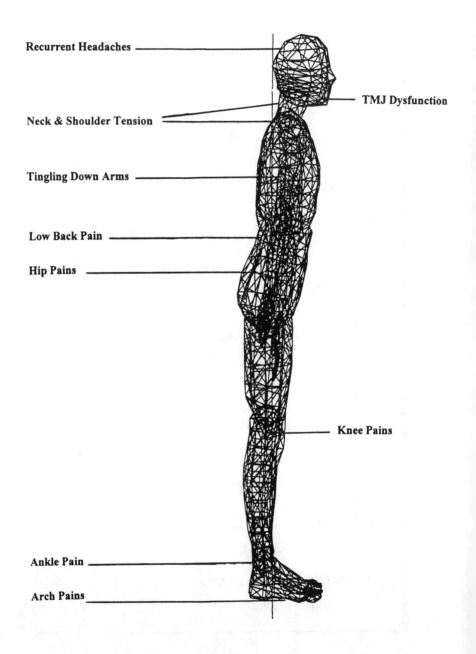

Recurrent Headaches

TMJ Dysfunction

Neck & Shoulder Tension

Tingling Down Arms

Low Back Pain

Hip Pains

Knee Pains

Ankle Pain

Arch Pains

Table of Contents

Part I – Background and Treatment

Part II – Case Histories

Part III - Self Help

Author's Note

There are words in this book that involve medical terminology. A Glossary has been provided at the end of the book, which I believe includes all those terms with which you may not be familiar.

Please, do not hesitate to use it.

You Are Not Alone

The number of people who suffer from postural pains/chronic pain syndromes foot to jaw is astounding. According to the National Center of Health Statistics, 112 million-plus people are so affected. There are millions more who suffer from acute episodes of postural pains for several months or longer. According to the U.S. Public Health Service reports, 80 million-plus people have had, or are presently suffering from, some form of painful back condition. Statistics have shown that 60% to 70% of people who have previously suffered back pain will have another bout of it within a two-year period. There are over 15 million people who are totally disabled by back pain. The financial impact for people suffering from and seeking medical care for this pain alone is staggering — approximately 60 billion dollars per year. These painful conditions also lead to limitations in lifestyles, which affect occupational capabilities and choices, physical fitness and sexual activities.

This book is about an important medical breakthrough in the understanding and treatment of such postural pains and chronic pain syndromes foot to jaw. For the first time, we are now able to identify the major, if not primary, cause of most of these problems. More importantly, we also know how to control the cause, so that we no longer just focus our attention on treating symptoms, but can actually get long-term resolution of the problems. This is done without the use of surgical or chemical intervention (drugs).

This medical breakthrough can help the millions of people suffering from these painful conditions physically, emotionally and financially. They can get better and stay that way, once and for all.

How I Lost My Pain

I had problems with my back and neck for years. For as long as I can remember, going back to my childhood, I never liked doing anything which required me to stand on my feet for long periods of time. I would get tired and irritable easily. I didn't realize until years later, while studying postural mechanics, that that wasn't normal.

As an adult, I have been bedridden for five to ten days at least four different times, over a fifteen year period. This is in addition to periodic episodes of pain in my legs, back, hips and neck, which did not require bed rest, but required a compromise of my lifestyle.

I had various types of treatment for my recurrent/chronic pains, ranging from oral anti-inflammatory medication and pain killers to physical therapy. I also had been given specific exercise programs to do regularly. In addition, I have had trigger point injections in my back and neck. I have had chiropractic manipulation and massage therapy. I have consulted an orthopedic surgeon and a physiatrist (physical medicine, rehabilitation specialist).

The result of all this is that I would get better after a few weeks or months and then go on for a while, until the next major episode.

As far as my professional life is concerned, I am a podiatrist and I have always had an interest in the biomechanical aspect of my field — that is, the study of how the foot, leg and skeletal system work to allow us to stand, walk, and run. It led me to realize that there were conservative, non-surgical alternatives to many foot and leg problems, and my practice reflected this attitude.

Over the years, I constantly sought out other practitioners who had similar interests. I found out that they were few and far between. However, my curiosity and persistence led me to a trip several years ago to Bellevue, Washington, where I had the opportunity to meet and subsequently train under Dr. Brian Rothbart.

Dr. Rothbart found that most people who suffer from recurrent postural pains/chronic pain syndromes foot to jaw are born with a specific weakness in their foot and leg structure. This weakness causes the foot to collapse. Because the body is connected from head to toe, and because humans exist on a planet with gravity, gravitational forces will produce mechanical strains on the body. Hence, when the foot collapses, the whole body can follow.

He then compared the human body's structure to that of a building. Just as the foundation of a building supports the superstructure, the foot

5

and ankle support the entire body. If the building's foundation weakens, it can collapse. Similarly, if the feet and ankles collapse, the whole body will follow, that is, will collapse also. This foot structural weakness is called forefoot varum.

By applying mechanical engineering principles, as related to building construction, to his already extensive knowledge of the human body's mechanics, Dr. Rothbart developed the science of "Posture Control Orthotic Therapy." This science enabled him to quantify the exact amount of excessive forefoot varum in each patient's feet. Furthermore, he was able to offset the negative effects of the foot's collapse and gravity by applying specific amounts of vertical force to the bottom of a patient's feet. He, with the help of Kathleen Yarrett, R.N., was able to do this by inventing "Posture Control Orthotics." The end result was that he was able to reduce and/or stop the foot's structural collapse. This, in turn, stabilized the skeletal structure and reversed the adverse effects (i.e., poor posture and recurrent postural pains/chronic pain syndromes foot to jaw) of this collapse on the entire body. Posture Control Orthotics (PCO®) has been granted a U.S. Patent number 5327664.

Clinically, Dr. Rothbart used this therapy on his patients and found that not only did their foot problems feel better, but often other musculoskeletal symptoms dramatically improved. Frequently, painful knees, hips, back, shoulder and neck problems started to resolve also.

I was in awe when I saw people with recurrent postural pains/chronic pain syndromes foot to jaw coming to him from all over the United States, including Alaska and Hawaii, and Canada.

In addition to teaching me all he had learned, Dr. Rothbart also treated me with Posture Control Orthotic Therapy. After years of recurrent episodes of leg, back and neck problems, my pains eventually totally receded. This was accomplished without any medications or surgical intervention.

Therefore, I made a commitment to myself that I would learn all I could about the therapy and use it in my own practice. In addition, I would try to disseminate this wonderful medical discovery to as many people as I could. Hence, one step towards this commitment is this book, *Nothing to lose . . . but the Pain.* It is about Posture Control Orthotic Therapy, which has been found to be extremely effective in reducing subjective symptoms associated with postural pains and chronic pain syndromes foot to jaw. More importantly, it has allowed for ongoing resolution of such pains. This is accomplished without surgery or drugs.

Acknowledgments

No one is an island. This book could not have been written without the assistance of several people. I would like to extend my personal gratitude to the following:

To my wife, Sharon Johnston Schneider, first for her endurance, patience and emotional support. Secondly, for her computer skills, critiquing, editing, research and writing abilities. She also named the book and designed the front and back covers. Finally, I would also like to thank her for her invaluable insights, and especially for her love and understanding.

Dr. Brian Rothbart, for creating Posture Control Orthotic Therapy, and teaching me all he knows so I may be able to help others. He also contributed information on two of the case histories.

Kathleen Yerratt, R.N., who, along with Dr. Rothbart, developed Posture Control Orthotics, and showed me how to use them to treat people with recurrent postural pains/chronic pain syndromes.

I would also like to thank Dr. Rothbart and Kathleen Yarratt, R.N. for letting me use the Subjective Outcome Studies that they had performed on chronic knee, back, and neck pain patients. These studies and their results appear in Appendix I of this book.

Mr. Will Mejia, for his unique, creative ability to turn my words into expert illustrations.

Finally, Mr. Alphons Hackl, president of Acropolis Books South, for his continued belief in me and my ideas.

Foreword

How It Helped Me
By Bernard E. Filner, M.D.

It is not often that a physician has the opportunity not only to introduce a new and improved treatment to benefit his patients, but that also plays a significant role in the treatment of his own condition. The introduction of a new type of device that is described by Dr. Schneider in this book, had a significant impact on the improved outcome in my treatment of both acute and chronic musculoskeletal conditions. In addition to the benefits that have accrued to my patients, my own neck and knee pain have markedly improved by utilizing these devices. There is no doubt in my mind that this approach will result in significant benefit to essentially any patient who is willing to make the commitment to using these devices properly, adjusting to them, and completing the process.

The concept that most people who develop chronic or recurring musculoskeletal pain have some underlying "perpetuating factor" that maintains these conditions and sets up circumstances for their recurrence, has been evolving in our treatment of these patients over the last ten to twenty years.

I have had the privilege of working with Dr. Schneider in managing these cases, and the results (including in my own case) have been remarkably and consistently good. Once the specific pain problem has been diagnosed and begun to be addressed, the underlying factors that lead to chronicity and recurrence need to be discovered and resolved. It appears as though the most "basic" perpetuating factor is the nature of the person's gait, and how their musculoskeletal system has adjusted to any abnormalities that were initially present. In its attempt to maintain balance and a reasonably upright erect posture, the body responds by what is known as a "bioimplosion" process, in which the muscles become exquisitely tight and inflexible in the major postural muscle groups. When subjected to injury, unless this musculature is allowed to "debrace," healing and the ultimate reconditioning and prevention of recurrence cannot occur. While it appears to be a relatively simple concept, it has not been adequately addressed until the present time.

8

A New Opportunity To Solve Problems
Before They Become Chronic

The other most important aspect of this approach is that it now gives us the opportunity to attempt to solve these problems before they become related to a chronic, recurring injury. If relatively "minor" sports injuries in youngsters are examined from this point of view, with a significant gait analysis, many of the later problems involving neck and back pain that people in their thirties through fifties experience could in all likelihood be mitigated or perhaps prevented. The cost implications to our national health care system would be enormous.

It is my hope that as you read this text, you will consider your own particular musculoskeletal difficulties, if they exist, and encourage you to further educate yourself, as well as investigate prevention and conservative treatment, rather than rushing to take medication or subject yourself to surgery. In addition, you, the consumer of medical care, can have a positive influence on the medical community to look more towards this type of preventive, conservative approach to resolving one of the greatest banes of our existence — chronic pain.

— Bernard E. Filner, M.D.

1

The Foot-To-Head Connection

As the song goes, the foot bone is connected to the ankle bone, the ankle bone is connected to the leg bone, and so on. There is no doubt that the entire body, from foot to head, is dynamically interrelated.

Actually, if you really think about it, the act of walking starts in our head. Our eyes focus on where we want to go, and a message gets transmitted through our brain, passing it down the body from the head, through the neck, spine, low back, legs and finally to our feet to start moving.

What actually gets us going is the body's falling forward. Walking is really repetitive acts of our body falling forward, and then one foot contacts the ground and we catch ourselves. In the meantime, the opposite foot and leg are moving off of the ground, getting ready to swing forward, thus causing us to fall forward again towards the next step. Man's bipedal mode of locomotion appears potentially catastrophic because only the rhythmic forward movement of the limbs keeps him from falling.

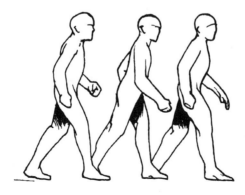

The foot, being the base of support for the body above, plays an important role in gait. First, it must be flexible, so it can absorb shock and adapt to whatever terrain we are walking on. Secondly, it must become rigid, to accept the body's weight from above and to withstand the propulsive force generated by the big toe pushing off against the ground.

Pronation and supination of the subtalar joint, the joint immediately below the ankle joint, give the foot this dual capability. This pronation unlocks the foot (makes it flexible), and supination of the subtalar joint, locks the foot (makes it rigid).

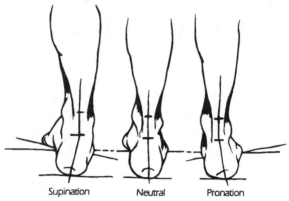

Supination   Neutral   Pronation

Pronation - Foot rolls inward and downward as the arch lowers a little. The leg rotates inward as well as the kneecap. This allows the foot to become flexible like "a loose bag of bones," to absorb shock and adapt to surfaces we walk on.
Supination - Foot rolls outward and upward as the arch rises. The leg and kneecap twist outwards. This allows the foot to become a very rigid, stable and strong platform. Needed to lift the weight of the body and move it forward.

The Gait Cycle

Normal walking, or gait, can best be understood by talking about the gait cycle. This is a series of movements that occurs within a certain period of time. One complete gait cycle starts when the heel of one's foot contacts the ground or walking surface and ends when the heel of the same foot contacts the ground or walking surface again. A series of gait cycles enables us to move from one location to another.

Normal Gait Cycle Right Foot and Leg

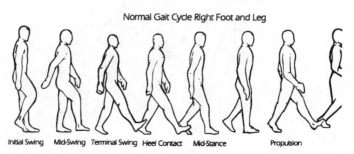

Initial Swing   Mid-Swing   Terminal Swing   Heel Contact   Mid-Stance   Propulsion

The Foot-To-Head Connection • 11

The typical gait cycle for each foot/leg is divided into two basic phases. The stance phase is 60% of the cycle, when the foot/leg is in contact with the ground; the swing phase, which is 40% of the gait cycle, is when the foot/leg is not in contact with the ground. It is moving, i.e., swinging; hence, the name swing phase.

There are also two brief periods when both feet/legs are in contact with the ground at the same time. This is called the double support phase, but for the purposes of this book, it need not be mentioned again.

The foot has three basic functions:

1. To absorb the shock of contact with the ground and help to dissipate this shock throughout the body.

2. To adapt to the surfaces on which we walk, run, dance, etc.

3. To accept the body weight from above and move it forward.

In order to accomplish this properly and on time, there is a series of three basic movements that each foot goes through. They are referred to as the three sub-phases of the stance phase of gait (i.e., when the foot is on the ground). They must occur in a set order and within a certain period of time. They are:

Heel contact – When the back part of the bottom of the foot contacts the ground.

Midstance – When the body's weight is moving over the middle of the foot.

Propulsion – When the weight is in the front of the foot and this part of the foot propels the body forward to the next step.

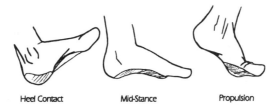

Heel Contact   Mid-Stance   Propulsion

The foot's ability to do what it has to do is directly related to a synchronized pattern of movements in the entire leg above it. Thus, at the beginning of heel contact, the hip is bent slightly (flexed) and rotated inward. The knee is straight (extended), the ankle is at a 90-degree angle with the ground, and the foot lands on the outside of its heel, at about a 4- to 6-degree angle to the ground. The foot then rolls inward and downward, as the arch lowers a little. The lower leg rotates

12

inward and the knee cap turns inward also. This series of motions is called pronation.

As this is occurring, the hip starts to become straighter (extends), the knee bends (flexes) and the foot starts to move downward against the ground at the ankle joint (plantar flexes). The entire lower leg is thus rotated inwardly, i.e., from the hip down. This allows the foot, upon heel contact, to become loose and mobile in order to do what it is supposed to do efficiently at this stage — absorb shock caused by the foot colliding with the ground (supporting surface) and allow the foot to adapt to whatever surface we are on, whether it be smooth, rough, level, unlevel, hard or soft. Thus, some amount of pronation is normal and necessary for smooth foot, leg and body function. The overall result of normal pronation is to allow the joints in the feet to be relatively loose or flexible, rather than restricted or tight.

After the foot has landed firmly and has started to bear the full weight of the body, the direction of the movement reverses. While the hip is still straight, the knee becomes straight, the foot starts to move upward towards the leg at the ankle joint (dorsiflexes), and though it is still in a pronated position, starts to also roll upward and outward. The arch starts to rise, and the kneecaps start to twist outward also. The foot is getting into a position so that it can be a very rigid, stable and strong platform needed to lift the weight of the body and move it forward. This series of motions is called supination. This is now known as the midstance phase, where most of the body's weight is centered in the middle of the foot. During this stage, the entire lower extremity from the hip down is rotated outward.

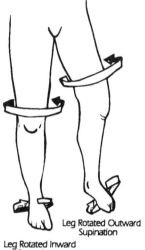

Leg Rotated Outward
Supination

Leg Rotated Inward
Pronation

The final stance phase is the propulsive phase, where the weight of the body is moved towards the toes, for toe-off. During the beginning of this propulsion phase, the hip is straight, the knee starts to bend, the foot starts to move downwards at the ankle joint and it remains in this very strong, supinated position. The lower extremity is still rotated outward.

Later on, in the propulsive stage, as the body weight gets set to be propelled off the large toe and on towards the next step, the hip starts to bend (flexes), the knee stays bent (flexed), the foot continues to move downward at the ankle joint (i.e., plantar flexes) and the foot stays in the supinated position until the last second, when it rolls in or pronates a little as the weight goes off the large toe. Again, the entire lower extremity is rotated outward.

Pronation - Supination

Stand up and rotate your right hip inwardly; the right leg will rotate in, and also the right foot will pronate, i.e., the ankle should roll inward and the arch should lower. This is pronation. Now do the opposite. Rotate your right hip outwards; the leg will rotate outward also, the ankle will turn outward and the arch will rise. This is supination.

Repeat the movements a few times and notice how much more loose and flexible the foot is when it is in the pronated position. Notice how much more stable and strong the foot is in the supinated position.

The Swing Phase

Now the foot is off the ground and is in the swing phase. This phase is the part of the gait cycle when the foot and the leg are non-weight-bearing and basically are moving forward. First, this phase allows the foot to clear the ground on the swing leg. Second, it also allows for this leg to move forward. It takes up about 40% of the gait cycle. It is divided into three subphases: the initial swing, mid-swing and terminal swing. Initial swing occurs at the beginning of swing phase when you have acceleration of movement, as the foot clears the ground and the leg moves forward. Then, when the swing leg is next to the leg on the ground, it is known as mid-swing. Finally, at the end of the swing phase (terminal swing), you have a slowing down or deceleration of the leg as it is preparing itself to make contact with the supportive surface.

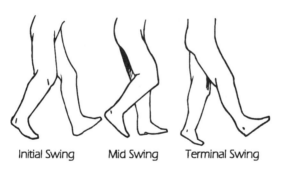

Initial Swing   Mid Swing   Terminal Swing

The Upper Body Involvement

The upper body also goes through its own sequences of motions to coincide and coordinate with those of the lower extremities. The part of the body which allows for this to occur is called the pelvis. The pelvis is the foundation of the spine. Therefore, the spine, back and the entire upper extremity all follow pelvic movements, and are thus interrelated with the gait cycle.

14

The pelvis is a ring of bones that form the hip region of the body. These are the sacrum, coccyx, ischium, ilium and the pubic bones. During walking, the pelvis goes through several different types of motions. It has a lateral, or side-to-side movement, which is necessary in order to keep the body's weight centered over the stance leg for balance. The pelvis also shifts up and down, i.e., it has a vertical movement. The high point usually occurs during the midstance of gait, and the low point is during heel contact. The purpose of this is to keep the center of gravity from not moving more than a few centimeters upward or downwards during walking. Finally, the pelvis can rotate a few degrees forward and backward. It usually swings forward on the swing leg and backward on the stance leg.

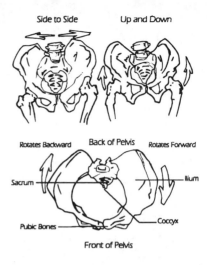

The chest area (thorax), i.e., the portion of the body that is above the diaphragm and below the neck, rotates in exactly the opposite direction of the pelvis. Therefore, as the pelvis rotates clockwise, the thorax will rotate counterclockwise. These rotations help regulate the speed at which a person walks.

As mentioned at the beginning of this chapter, walking is really a series of falling forward and stopping our falls. Our arms move forward and backwards in order to balance out our forward fall, and they also help create motion or energy to fuel our walking. As one's hip swings forward, the opposite arm also swings forward.

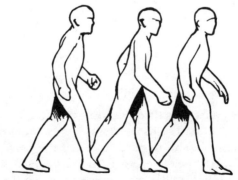

As one hip swings forward, the opposite arm swings forward

Our upper body also tilts forward a little at the chest area. The neck and head are attached to the upper body, and, therefore, they will also be thrust forward at this time. If we change directions in walking, we have to turn our neck and turn our head, rotate our shoulders and the rest of the body will follow.

Excessive Pronation and Musculoskeletal Problems

Timing is extremely important. If the joints and the muscles are working efficiently and smoothly in the lower extremities, then the foot is able to go from pronation to supination smoothly and on time, with no strain or loss of efficient motion. If someone excessively pronates, the weight of the body falls on the foot at the wrong time. Instead of being able to be a rigid, stable structure, the foot is often a "loose bag of bones," and cannot possibly propel the body forward efficiently. Instead of being in a strong supinated position, it is often in a pronated or weakened state. As we have seen, the foot bone is connected to the ankle bone, the ankle bone is connected to the leg bone, and so on. Hence, this can cause many postural pains foot to jaw.

Muscles which are designed for stabilization are called upon to propel; propeller muscles are forced to help with stabilization. When the various muscle groups in our body are called upon to do work that they were not intended to do, they become strained, and performance levels are diminished. The body may also start to collapse, so to speak. Another problem occurs because the body weight is thrust on the foot at a time when it is unstable. The bones are subjected to abnormal stresses, which can lead to stress fractures, bone spur formations, enlargement of bones called exostoses, joint injuries, bursitis and degenerative arthritis. When the muscles are forced to do the wrong work, as described above, stresses are created, which can lead to muscle and tendon injuries. Excessive stresses are often transmitted through the legs to the skeletal structure, producing many of the knee, hip, back, shoulder, neck and facial area postural pains/chronic pain syndromes that we see.

2

What Causes Pain?

*The Cause of Most Postural Pain
And Chronic Pain Syndromes*

Scientific Background

It's a medical fact that much of the pain in your back, hips, legs, knees and ankles is caused by your feet. Why? Because if your feet are not properly aligned, and most people's are not, undue stress is placed on all the muscles, joints and bones of your body. The result: Your feet may not hurt at all, but your joints, bones, tendons and muscles from foot to jaw may be in serious trouble. Studies have shown that inefficient foot and leg functioning often leads to various recurrent and chronic postural pains.

Unfortunately, because of evolutionary failure, most of us are born with a tendency towards inefficient foot and leg functioning. As a result, the front of the inside of one's foot is actually angled off the ground an excessive number of degrees when one's foot actually contacts the ground to walk.

The problem actually starts in the developing fetus. As the lower extremity (foot and leg) begins to develop, the inner border of the front of the foot is twisted inward and upward, from the mid-line (middle of the body) a certain amount of degrees. During the fourth month of development, the head and neck of one of the larger bones in the back of

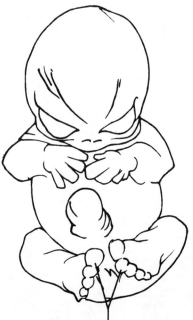

Inner border of front of foot
twisted inward and upward

the foot, called the talus, is supposed to twist outward and downward. The front of the foot follows this movement, and when we are born, the inner border of the front of the foot should still be twisted inward and upward approximately four to six degrees from the mid-line of the body. When we begin to walk, the inner portion of the foot, including the front of the foot and large toe joint, must be brought down in order to contact the ground for shock absorption, balance, support and for propelling us forward to the next step.

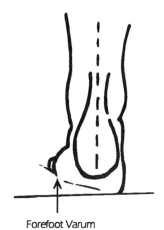

Forefoot Varum

However, in many of us, this outward and downward derotation of the foot fails to completely occur in the fetus. Thus, the inner border of the front of the foot is elevated or twisted inward and upward a greater amount of degrees than is considered ideal for normal, efficient standing/walking. This is called excessive forefoot varum. Because of this, the foot is forced to roll inward and downward excessively (collapses) in order for the total foot to reach the ground, which is necessary to walk. This is called excessive pronation.

This inefficient foot and leg functioning is usually not unsightly or obvious to the average person. Professionals who are trained to evaluate body biomechanics and gait (walking) analysis are best qualified to determine the degree of inefficient body mechanics.

The Role of Gravity

Most of us take gravity for granted. We know that it allows us to maintain contact with the ground and to walk by using the ground for propulsion. What we frequently forget is that gravity is also a constant force which tries to push us downward into the ground.

When man became erect, he challenged gravity with his upright posture. Instead of distributing the force of gravity on two hands and two feet, he doubled the effect of gravity on his spine and lower extremities by becoming bipedal. The resultant increase in pressure on his skeletal structures tends to magnify any weakness (such as excessive pronation) over a period of years.

We associate youth with a straight, upright posture. Conversely, we picture the elderly as being stooped and possibly requiring a cane for additional support. This typifies the advanced changes caused by gravitational forces. The degenerative process, wherein we gradually lose our erect posture, has been called "postural collapse."

The Cause of Postural Collapse

Because the body is connected from head to toe, what affects one part of the body affects every other part. This is called the compensatory concept of motion. Because humans exist on a planet with gravity, gravitational stress produces mechanical strains on the body when the foot collapses. This collapse represents an unstable foundation for the superstructure (the body above). Subsequently, the whole body follows it, i.e., the whole body starts to collapse. Again, this is something that is not always readily apparent to the average person.

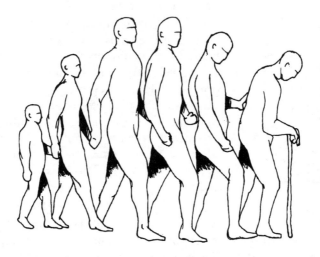

There are five skeletal system changes that we note during postural collapse. These occur in stages and may not be obvious in all cases. First, there is excessive pronation of the feet, which is visually seen as a rolling inward and downward of the feet because the front of the foot is off the ground an excessive amount of degrees. The arch may be high, average or flat. Secondly, as the center of gravity is shifted from the center of the feet to the inside of the feet, the knees are forced inward and closer together. This is called Genu Valgum (knock-kneed). Third of all, the sacroiliac joint, located in the low back area, then rotates forward and downward (swayback); thus, you have a forward rotation of the hips. The collapsing foot drives the pelvis forward as the body's center of gravity is anterior to or in front of the sacroiliac joint. This pelvic rotation carries the lumbar spine, i.e., the back, with it, producing Lumbar Lordosis, or forward

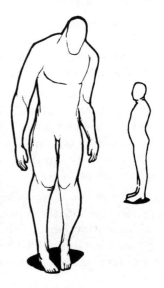

curvature of the lumbar spine in the low back. This leads to a compensatory, inward rotation of the upper back, or Thoracic Kyphosis, seen visually as "swayback" and "hunched shoulders." Finally, this causes the cervical (neck) spine to lose its normal curvature, and the head is thrust forward. The end result is a postural collapse, inward and forward, foot to jaw.

An appropriate analogy would be to compare what we have discussed to a building's structure. If a building has a weak foundation, it will have problems and could eventually collapse. Such a building might initially have some of the following problems, which are often recurrent if the foundation is not fixed: The front door constantly jams, there are cracks in the walls on the second and third floors, the shingles get loose and fall off from the roof. You have these problems fixed, and, a few years later, you notice one or more of them recurring or new ones occurring, and you have them fixed again. Finally, you realize that your building continues to have problems because it has a weak foundation. Until you fix the foundation, you will constantly be fixing the problems and not addressing the actual cause.

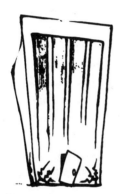 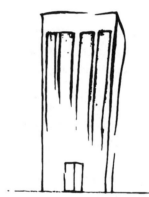

Well, this is the same thing with the human body and postural collapse. With postural collapse, the weak foundation is your feet; the front door jamming could be leg and knee pains. Second and third floor cracking could be low back area problems, and the shingles falling off the roof can be your neck and head aches.

The Consequences of Postural Collapse

Since this collapse places the body in an unstable and inefficient functioning position, the muscles in the body follow this collapse, with the following results: Muscles on the inside of the legs are constantly stretched and strained; the muscles on the outside of the legs are contracted or shortened. In addition, muscles on the front of the upper body are contracted, or tight. The muscles in the back of the body, in general, especially the upper body, are stretched or lengthened. Thus, many of the skeletal system's muscles in the body are either too tight and under too much tension, or stretched too much and are too weak. This leads to postural pain/chronic pain syndromes foot to jaw.

Muscles are attached to tendons, which are attached to bone; two or more bones make up a joint. Therefore, we can see how such abnormal muscle stress can lead to joint and bone changes and painful conditions such as degenerative joint diseases, arthritis, bursitis, joint injuries and bone spur formations. Muscles that are constantly being stressed can lead to muscle cramps, spasms, aches, pains and injuries. Nerves can be compressed and injured, causing diminished sensations, numbness and painful conditions. Tendons and ligaments (soft tissue which attaches bone to bone) also can become strained, sprained and injured.

Other Things To Consider

As we can see, it is obvious that there is a dynamic interrelationship from the feet to legs, the legs to the pelvis (hip), and pelvis to the spine (back) and above. Hence, any imbalance or malalignment of the feet that leads to faulty foot function will usually have a profound and negative effect on the body above. In addition to this, here are some other important facts to ponder:

1. One half of the body's 650 muscles are involved in walking, running, or any fitness activities.

2. Though our feet represent only a small fraction of our body's weight, they are expected to support, balance and move the remainder of our body's weight smoothly and efficiently.

3. The average person takes approximately 7,000 footsteps per day and walks approximately 115,000 miles in a lifetime.

4. Fitness activities can increase the body's weight, and therefore increase stress on each foot and lower extremity from 2 to 3½ times of what it normally is.

It is, therefore, no wonder that if there is even a minor foot and leg structural weakness, imbalance or imperfection, postural pain/chronic pain syndromes can occur.

We Are Unique Individuals

It is important to note that although most of us are born with inefficient foot and leg functioning due to excessive pronation, and not everybody exhibits painful skeletal conditions, some of us unfortunately, develop chronic pains and others have episodes that lay them up for short periods of time.

The reason for this is that we are unique individuals. There are varying degrees of excessive pronation ranging from mild to severe. Obviously, those of us who only have mild excessive pronation are not going to have the kinds of problems, in most cases, that someone with moderate or severe pronation will have. In addition, the kinds of lifestyles that we lead can have a definite effect on the wear and tear of our bodies. Someone who has excessive pronation and is an athlete is likely to have more problems from overuse than someone who has a sedentary lifestyle and is relatively non-athletic. A person who takes care of his body and is careful with diet, weight, appropriate exercises and type of shoes is more likely to be better able to withstand the negative effects of excessive pronation, as well as other health problems.

In addition, there are billions of people on this earth, and hardly any of us look exactly alike. None of our bodies is exactly the same, though we have the same amount of muscles, bones and joints.

The Effects of Trauma

As we have already seen, someone who has excessive pronation will be walking, standing, and running at a distinct disadvantage, mechanically speaking. Therefore, it is more likely that that person will suffer from postural pain/chronic pain syndromes. Though this does not represent direct trauma, it is subtle trauma. People who are fitness enthusiasts and are unfortunately endowed with a weak structure will be more likely to get overuse/fitness injuries. Not only that, it will be more difficult, or impossible, for some of these people to fully overcome these injuries for any long period of time. Many of these people will say that they took a month or two off and that as soon as they built back up to a certain level of activity, the injury recurred. This is because their body had been functioning with very tense muscles, which were working along improper fulcrums; the bones and joints in the body were essentially in a malaligned position. Therefore, it is the postural collapse, due to excessive forefoot varum and excessive pronation, that is the culprit that is often overlooked. These people often have symptoms treated, but not the real cause.

Obviously, people who have suffered severe trauma, such as a fall, or a bad car accident, are more prone to have chronic pains throughout their lifetime. What is often overlooked and misunderstood is that these people also pronate excessively; their musculoskeletal systems have been overworked already in trying to compensate for it and prevent the postural collapse for years. Hence, their muscles and bodies have been under constant physical stress, and they often cannot rebound from the traumatic event.

Finally, some people undergo musculoskeletal system surgery for one reason or another. This is traumatic. Some of us recover better than others, and one of these reasons could be the fact that if a person has excessive pronation, his body is constantly under stress, and is unable to heal effectively.

3

What Postural Problems Are We Talking About?

Foot/Heel Pains

Bunions

A bunion is a bone enlargement and/or swelling which can occur either on the outside of the big toe joint or the outside of the little toe joint. Along with a bunion, your foot maybe misshapen — the big toe turning in towards the other toes. The condition can get progressively worse and can lead to more degenerative changes.

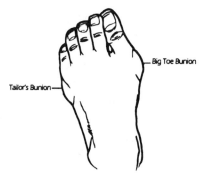

The small toe joint bunion, or Tailor's bunion, is an enlargement of the outside of the head of the fifth metatarsal bone. This is the bone directly behind the fifth (little) toe.

Hammertoes

Hammertoes are contracted, claw-like toes, which are often due to a muscle imbalance. This causes the toes to buckle and become hammered in appearance.

Corns and Calluses

Corns and calluses are abnormal thickening of the skin, which results from friction and pressure under or over a boney area. Corns are usually found on tops of the toes. Occasionally, some corns occur in between two adjacent toes. These are called soft corns and are often extremely painful.

Calluses are a buildup of thickened skin, which usually occurs in areas of extreme friction and pressure, such as those under the boney areas of the ball of the feet.

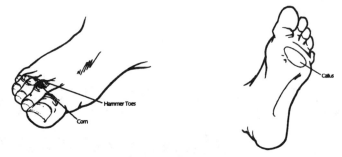

Neuroma

A neuroma is a nerve tumor in the front of the foot. This irritates the nerves and causes them to enlarge. This is usually associated with a burning, stinging, or knife-like pain in adjacent toes.

Metatarsalgia

Pain located within the second, third, fourth, and occasionally the fifth metatarsophalangeal joints (the joints behind the second, third, fourth and fifth toes respectively) is called metatarsalgia.

Sesamoiditis

There is an area behind the big toe, under the inside of the bottom of the foot, that can often get irritated and painful. The condition is called sesamoiditis because the pain is located under two small bones in this area, called the sesamoid bones.

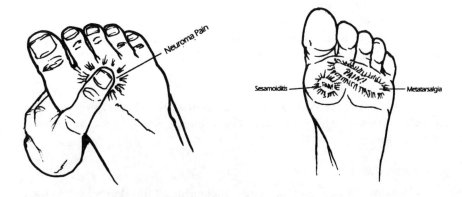

Foot Stress Fractures

Stress fractures in the foot most commonly occur in the metatarsal bones (the bones behind the four lesser toes), but occasionally can affect the metatarsal bone behind the large toe. These are small cracks in the bone that are often due to overuse and excessive pronation.

Heel and Arch Pain

There are several causes of heel and arch pain, such as bone spurs, soft tissue inflammation, or a strain of the long plantar ligament on the bottom of the foot (plantar fascia), extending from the back of the heel, through the arch, to the front of the foot and ending behind the toes, called plantar fasciitis.

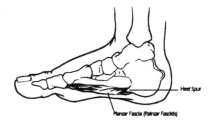

Apophysitis

This is a painful condition that occurs in young people between the ages of 8 and 15. The pain is located at the back and bottom of the heel. It is an irritation of the growth plate (cartilage) in the back of the calcaneus or heel bone.

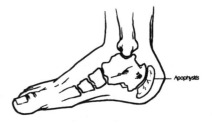

Chronic Ankle Instability and Pain

This is a condition that occurs in people who are prone to have multiple and recurrent ankle sprains. Also, this condition occurs because initial or previous ankle sprains were never allowed to heal properly. The most common area of the ankle that is involved is the outside of the ankle.

There are other painful ankle conditions, such as tendinitis, which is an inflammation of a tendon, often on the inside of the ankle. In addition, there are ankle joint changes such as bone spurs, which can form on the talus bone in the front of the ankle joint. This decreases the space in the joint and can lead to painful conditions.

Pain on the inside or medial side of the ankle joint can be due to a strained ligament, inflammation of a tendon or an entrapped nerve, called the Tarsal Tunnel Syndrome.

The Lower Leg

Problems in the lower leg are usually due to muscle strains and inflammation of the tendons.

The calf muscle inserts or ends in the Achilles tendon in the back lower aspect of the leg, and often this tendon can become inflamed, swollen and painful. This is commonly known as Achilles tendinitis.

Shin splints is an all-purpose term used to describe problems in the front and inside parts of the lower leg. These usually are brought on by fitness activities, but can occur with prolonged walking also.

Stress fractures are minute cracks in the bones of the lower legs. They are due to overuse and overstress, and are often related to excessive foot pronation.

Finally, the muscles in the lower legs sometimes go into painful spasms. This usually occurs in the powerful calf muscles in the back of the lower legs.

Knee Pains

Tendinitis

Tendinitis is inflammation of any of the tendons surrounding the knee joint. The most common one ends just below the knee cap in the front upper portion of the lower leg.

You can also get tendinitis at the origin of the calf muscles in the back area of the knee, as well as the hamstring tendons. The hamstrings are the muscles in the back of the thigh and they can become strained (hamstring pull).

Bursitis

Bursitis can also occur around the knee joint. The knee has several bursal sacs, which are fluid filled sacs that are used to lubricate various spaces around joints. These sacs can sometimes become irritated and inflamed from excessive stress.

Chondromalacia Patella

Chondromalacia patella is a term that is commonly used. It has to do with irregularities, irritation and disintegration of the back of the kneecap, or patella.

Past Knee Injuries

Past knee injuries, such as ligament injuries due to trauma such as football injuries, can often lead to very unstable, weak and painful knees. Inefficient foot and leg functioning, i.e., excessive pronation, just compounds the instability and pains associated with this. Often the instability is present because the original injury was not treated properly, i.e., undertreated, the patient did not listen to doctor recommendations, or it was improperly rehabilitated. This can also lead to degenerative or osteoarthritis of the knees.

Knee Sprain

Knee sprain is an injury which is due to a ligament that gets sprained or stressed in the knee.

Osgood-Schlatter's Disease

Osgood-Schlatter's disease produces pain in front of and just below the knee joint. This is due to an irritation and fragmentation of a bone in the lower leg called the tibia. This usually occurs in boys between the ages of 9 and 14 years.

Thigh Injuries

Injuries in the thigh area usually involve the muscles and tendons. Inflammation of the muscle is called myositis; inflammation of the tendon is called tendinitis. Muscles can also be strained or pulled. The most common muscle group involved is the hamstring in the back of the thighs.

Painful muscle spasms can also occur in this area. Occasionally, stress fractures occur in the thigh bone (femur), usually related to fitness activities.

Finally, the tensor fascia latae muscle, which originates on the outside of the buttocks and upper thigh area, can get strained, tight, and/or irritated. This muscle inserts (ends) in the illiotibial band on the outside of the thigh, and itself ends just below the outside of the knee joint. Pains at the insertion of this band at the outside of the knee joint are often due to an irritated tendon from the tensor fascia latae muscle above. This is called the tensor fascia latae illiotibial band syndrome.

Hip

Painful conditions around the hip include: Degenerative arthritis (hip joint inflammation), bursitis (inflammation of the bursal sac in the hip joint) and capsulitis (inflammation of the thick fibrous capsule around the hip joint).

Muscular injuries in the thigh or low back can also cause hip joint stiffness and pains.

Hip and Knee Joint Replacements

Unfortunately, some people who suffer from chronic hip and knee pains have to undergo hip and knee joint replacement surgery. Apparently, there has been sufficient damage through direct trauma, degenerative joint disease and/or infection to these joints that they require such a procedure.

Back Pains

Back pain, as many of us know, can wreak havoc with your lifestyle. Many people assume back pain is almost a normal part of life, because it is so prevalent. It is usually not caused by just one incident or injury. It is, frequently, the result of years of poor posture, bad biomechanics, stress of living and working habits, loss of flexibility and lack of overall physical conditioning. Major problems associated with mechanical back pain include degenerative disc disease. This occurs from years of wear and tear on the discs in your spinal cord, which may be associated with poor posture and/or utilizing your back in a precarious position. Major injuries such as car accidents or falls can lead to this. There are also certain congenital conditions you are born with, such as curvature of the spine, called scoliosis or spondylolisthesis, which is a forward misalignment of a vertebra or an underdeveloped vertebra called a hemi-vertebra.

Muscle spasms and strains in the low back area are extremely common, as are joint problems, especially in the sacroiliac joint in the lower back area.

Sciatica

Sciatica is pain that runs along the course of the sciatic nerve. This is usually due to an injury or inflammation to the nerve or its root. The pain goes from the buttocks, radiating down the back of the thigh and calf. There can also be tenderness, tingling and numbness along the nerve.

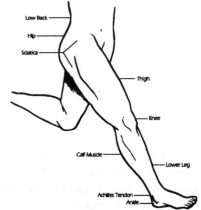

Thoracic Outlet Syndrome

Thoracic outlet syndrome is usually a complex symptom due to compression of a nerve on one side of the neck, and is usually characterized by pain and/or numbness in the hand on that side of the body, especially the fourth and fifth fingers, and sometimes the forearm.

Occasionally, the vein or lymph nodes get compressed, and swelling of the fingers and top of the hand occurs.

Shoulder Pains

Shoulder pains can be due to an inflammation of the fluid sacs in your shoulder called the bursa. This is called bursitis. An inflammation of the tendons around the shoulder area is called tendinitis. Also, degenerative arthritis can occur in the shoulder joint. Nerves that are pinched or compressed in the neck can cause pain in the shoulder area, again radiating down the arm.

TMJ
Neck Pains
Shoulder Pains
Thoracic Outlet Syndrome

Neck Pains

Pains in the neck are extremely common. This is because the neck is easily injured; it also gets a lot of abuse and wear and tear. The major symptom of neck problems is a stiff neck, where there is a lack of motion in the neck. This can lead to chronic headaches.

Whiplash, which is often associated with car and sports injuries, occurs when the neck area sustains a severe jarring. It literally snaps or is jarred backwards. It can then become sprained and injured. Degenerative joint disease can occur in the various cervical discs in the neck. Nerves can also get pinched or irritated in the neck area. This can lead to pain radiating down your arm, all the way to your hand.

Transmandibular Joint Dysfunction (TMJ)

This is a well-known orthopedic dental problem which often has very painful symptoms ranging from headaches and chronic sinus conditions to neck and shoulder pain, pain radiating down the arms and back pain.

Some people often experience grinding in their teeth at night. Tenderness in the facial muscles and clicking are often noted. A limitation of movement or an irregular tracking pattern of the jaw bone is often present. With TMJ, you also can have an abnormal bite, where one side of the jaw is higher than the other. This causes muscles in the facial area to go into spasm.

Degenerative Joint Disease

Excessive pronation produces eccentric erosion patterns in weight-bearing joints. Clinically, these joint changes are termed osteo-degenerative arthritis.

Cartilage is elastic, semi-hard tissue that covers some bones and particularly joint surfaces. It allows for smooth motion and diminishes friction in the joint. If the joint is damaged, then the two opposing surfaces will become rough and irregular. There is a loss of cartilage and the joint itself often becomes narrowed. This is referred to as degenerative arthritis. Most people eventually develop some form of degenerative arthritis, but some people are more predisposed than others. In some of these people, this can result in severe pain and disability. Abnormal or excessive stress on the joint, either by direct trauma or subtle trauma, due to abnormal tracking patterns in the joint, is one of the primary causes of degenerative arthritis. Hence, excessive pronation which leads to postural collapse, which we have already discussed, can certainly be a major factor in contributing to this very prevalent and painful condition.

Degenerative arthritis can occur in any major joint in the body, but is often very prevalent in the knees, hips and shoulders, as well as the bones in the spinal cord.

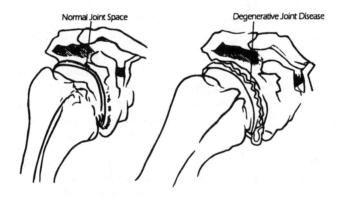

Normal Joint Space   Degenerative Joint Disease

Fibromyalgia

Fibromyalgia is a condition of general muscular aches and pains that hurt all the time. It most often affects the neck, shoulders and hip. It is believed to be caused by muscle stress, tension, trauma or illness. Muscles can often remain tense and achy all day long. They are also stiff, and movement becomes difficult. The pain is often present whether you are up moving around or sitting still, or even trying to sleep.

Myofascial Syndrome

Myofascial syndrome, pain in one part of the body caused by an injury or an irritation to a muscle at a different location (pain felt elsewhere than at its true site), is termed "referred pain." For example, tightness in the neck muscles can lead to radiating pain down your arm. Another example is you can have very tight or strained neck muscles that cause headaches. You can have a pain in your foot which is caused by an irritated muscle in the lower leg; for instance, chronic or recurrent heel pain can be caused by tightness in a calf muscle.

Pregnancy and Low Back Pain

Frequently, pregnant women suffer with low back pains. This is due in part to the enlarged abdomen, which produces strain on the lower back muscles. In addition, if a person is an excessive foot pronator, these symptoms will be even more exacerbated. PCO therapy has been found to be very effective in dealing with this painful condition. See Chapter 18 "Pregnancy and Postural Pains."

Recurrent/Overuse Sports Injuries

Sports, fitness and dance activities, unfortunately, often lead to a variety of what are termed overuse injuries. Some of the more common injuries include heel pain and plantar fasciitis, recurrent ankle sprains/pains, Achilles tendinitis, calf strains, shin splints, stress fractures in the lower leg and metatarsal bones of the feet. This also includes various knee injuries and recurrent knee problems such as patella tendinitis, femoral patella stress syndrome, chondromalacia of the knee, bursitis of the knee, and illiotibial band syndrome. In addition, there are hip bursitis, hamstring, groin, lower back, upper back, neck, and shoulder strains and pains.

Chronic Pain Syndromes

Chronic pain syndrome patients are people who experience long-term, unrelenting pain in various parts of their body, from the feet to the legs, knees, hips, back, neck, shoulder, jaw and head. The typical scenario for these patients is they get various types of treatments, such as manual medicine, physical therapy, oral anti-inflammatory medication, muscle relaxants, painkillers, steroid injections, and trigger point injections. Many are referred for psychotherapy, given anti-depressants, nutritional counseling or weight control. Often, one or combinations of these therapies work, but for short periods of time. Most patients feel and get better to some extent *as long as they remain in therapy.*

Frustration level with this scenario rises when a patient goes out of therapy. Sometime later, they have to come back for more care, and tell you they feel even worse. What happens is a cycle of relentless, chronic pain that gets worse and worse as time goes on. They get better with care, leave care, get worse again, come back for more care. However, their symptoms seem worse, and they do not get as better as before. They leave therapy and drop down even further. There is a cycle downward. This is the "Chronic Pain Syndrome."

What also compounds the frustration is that a patient often goes to a different doctor because nothing has really worked or helped them. So a single doctor or medical professional is often not tracking the patient, observing that he is getting worse and worse.

4

The Solution: Posture Control Orthotic Therapy

P osture Control Orthotic Therapy has been found to be extremely effective in reducing subjective symptoms associated with postural pain/chronic pain syndromes foot to jaw. More importantly, it has allowed for ongoing resolution of such pains.

The goal of Posture Control Orthotic Therapy is to compensate for excessive pronation which leads to postural pains and/or postural collapse.

The Treatment Process

Process Control Orthotic Therapy is actually a process. First, a detailed history and physical examination are performed. This is done in order to quantify the amount of excessive pronation that a patient exhibits, how the body has compensated for it and has been negatively affected by it. An evaluation of all weight-bearing joints, muscle testing and gait analysis are all important components of the exam.

In addition to excessive pronation, various other factors that can perpetuate postural pains are identified. This includes how you sit, stand, work, sleep, weight, nutritional needs, shoe wear, and fitness activities, etc.

From all the information gathered above, an individualized treatment program is established for each patient.

1. Posture Control Orthotics are utilized to control excessive pronation. They are prescriptive orthotics, specifically designed for patients with acute and chronic postural pains.

2. Individualized exercise programs may be recommended.

3. How to eliminate, minimize or compensate for other perpetuating factors are identified and discussed.

Posture Control Orthotic Stage Therapy

By gradually decreasing excessive pronation patterns of feet, negative skeletal system changes can be compromised and/or reversed. This is done in a series of incremental orthotic changes (Posture Control Orthotic State Therapy), where vertical lift is gradually applied to the inside ball of the foot, through a device called a Posture Control Orthotic, to increase foot-to-ground contact. Vertical ground forces are gradually applied to the body's foundation, i.e., under the feet, to offset excessive pronation and the gravitational forces coming down. By utilizing these orthotics, a patient is put into a position where he is structurally more stable. The abnormal muscle tension, and patterns that have developed because of this, are now able to unwind.

The results of mechanical dysfunction, which has led to recurrent postural pain/chronic pain syndromes and/or postural collapse, take years to develop. The body has to be given time to gradually bring itself back to vertical. Thus, incremental changes are necessary to give the body an opportunity to adapt to the changes with as little reaction as possible. This allows us to get a gradual unwinding of the posture from foot to jaw. As we increase the vertical height, the symptoms start to resolve, usually from the ground up. This is done by a technique called posting or shimming (building the ground up to the foot). Intolerance can occur if these incremental changes in posting are too aggressive. It is the same precaution that an orthodontist follows when straightening teeth.

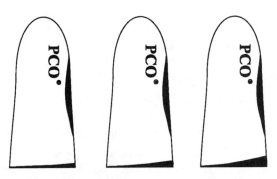

Postural Control Orthotics   Incremental Changes

Posture Control Orthotic Therapy gradually increases foot stability, decreases excessive pronation, reverses postural collapse and allows the body to become more erect or vertical. The closer to vertical, the more linearly the joints of the body will track. The body will function more efficiently, feel better and heal. The first pair of orthotics will be dispensed a few weeks after the doctor has prescribed them.

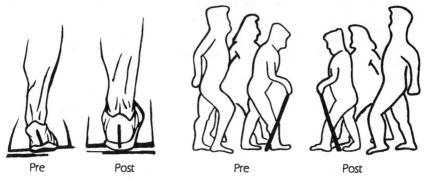

| Pre | Post | Pre | Post |

Posture Control Orthotic Therapy

Several pairs of Posture Control Orthotics are often needed, depending upon the severity of the excessive pronation. This is because the muscles need time to unwind. As they do, the structure of the body changes. Using PCOs is a time-oriented process. Healing is cyclical. If adjustments are too severe, inflammatory reactions may occur. If adjusted gradually, beneficial effects are noted.

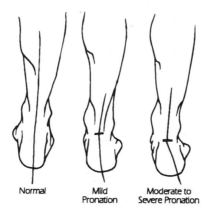

| Normal | Mild Pronation | Moderate to Severe Pronation |

Pain Storm

After an initial break-in period, the patient should be able to wear the PCOs all of the time. Soon a reduction or elimination of some, or even all, of the symptoms will be reported, usually from the ground up.

After a period of time, usually around three months or so, some or all of the symptoms may start to recur, or a new one is felt. This is called pain storming. What has happened is the unwinding of muscles that had been collapsing. In other words, as the muscles start to realign themselves and relax, the body unwinds and the symptoms start to recede. However, after a period of time, the angle of the foot and leg to the ground changes. In addition, the contour and shape of the foot may change, so that the Posture Control Orthotic no longer fits properly. Nor will it control your body's mechanics as it did originally. This means you are in need of more biomechanical control, i.e., more wedging. This is why several pairs of orthotics are often needed.

Temps

Temps, wedges or posts all stand for material that is applied to the underside of a Posture Control Orthotic to increase the supportive/controlling effect of the device upon the foot and body. They are two millimeters in thickness. When a person experiences a pain storm, excessive pronation measurements are retaken. As the muscles in the body unwind, excessive pronation measurements will increase. Therefore, more control, i.e., vertical lift, is needed to offset this change. Temporary posts or wedges are then applied to the inside part of the bottom of the existing orthotic. This is done to give more support in order to temporarily stop the pain storm while the next pair of orthotics, with a new prescription, is being made. It also helps ascertain how much more control the patient needs and can tolerate. This new pair will be dispensed in approximately two to four weeks.

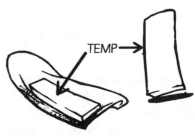

TEMP attached to PCO

The Final Pair

After several pairs, you will finally receive your last pair, which is the highest posting that is going to be needed to control your excessive pronation. This pair is reached when pain storms no longer occur. At this time, you will be discharged from immediate care. If you start to experience another pain storm, you will need a new pair of PCOs. This is usually due to a breakdown of the materials the orthotic is made of. It is recommended that yearly visits be established to try and prevent this from occurring.

Contraindications

Posture Control Orthotic Therapy is not for all patients, especially those who exhibit the following symptoms:

1. Boney fusions, such as: triple arthrodesis, spinal fusions, boney ankle equinus.
2. Tumor/cancer.
3. Infections.

4. Invasive arthritis, such as psoriatic dermatitis, ankylosing spondylitis, infectious or septic polyarthritic conditions.

5. Severe psychological dysfunction.

6. Limited range of motion, very tight muscles.

7. Rigidity, no flexibility.

Age

Age is not as important a factor, although, in general, it becomes more difficult to adjust postural mechanics as one gets older. This means you have to be very determined to go through it at an older age. For the same reasons, an orthodontist or dentist will tell you it is easier to move teeth around at twelve than at fifty, but it still can be done. It will just take longer, probably be more painful and more resistant. If someone is committed to doing it, and motivated enough, it can be accomplished. It depends on the patient's determination. As a rule, patients between the ages of 10 and 70 do well with Posture Control Orthotic Therapy.

Things to Consider – This Is Not a Quick Fix

1. It can take 12 to 18 months and 3 to 5 pairs of Posture Control Orthotics in some cases.

2. The orthotics may be uncomfortable at times, usually only during the break-in period. Like orthodonture work, a new pair of Posture Control Orthotics often hurts for a few days or weeks. It will sometimes feel like there is a rock under the arch of the foot. But as the first week or two of the break-in period goes by, your feet will start to feel much better. Then your symptoms, from your feet upwards, will start to respond.

3. There are going to be some restrictions on the types of shoes that can be worn.

4. The orthotics must be worn at least 70% of the time to really have positive results.

5. Occasionally, other health care professionals are needed in this process.

Expectations

While Posture Control Orthotic Therapy has been very successful in treating postural pains foot to jaw, that doesn't necessarily mean that a person is going to get 100% elimination of every symptom. Remember, many people needing this type of treatment have multiple symptoms, their pain has been ongoing for years, and they may have had trauma or multiple doctors. What a person can reasonably expect is a diminishing of their symptoms, if not a total recession of them.

In some cases, any reduction of the symptoms would be welcome. For example, if someone is unable to work and has chronic pains in several areas of his body, and pain can be diminished to the point where that person is able to work and be on his feet for a full or even a half day, that is considered a successful treatment. If a person has ongoing pain and is fifty to sixty years old, he may feel 100% better. But if his expectations are that he is going to be able to do certain activities that he did when he was twenty to thirty, that is not realistic.

If a person has had chronic postural pains for long periods of time and has had success using Posture Control Orthotics, it still means there may be certain limitations in activities such as lifting.

Postural Control Orthotics vs. Arch Supports and Conventional Orthotics

Posture Control Orthotics have been granted a U.S. patent #5327664.

Excessive pronation can be controlled, allowing the feet, legs and skeletal system to function normally and with maximum efficiency. This can be effectively done by utilizing Posture Control Orthotic Therapy. Posture Control Orthotics are custom-made orthotics, form fitted to each patient's feet. PCOs can actually change the postural mechanics from foot to jaw. They apply a force to the bottom of the foot which is much more efficient in point and vertical correction application than anything that preceded them.

As we have explained, the cause of most postural pains foot to jaw and chronic pain syndromes is excessive pronation (due to forefoot varum), which is a congenital/inherited trait, whereby the inside of the front of the foot is twisted off the ground an excessive amount of millimeters or degrees. This makes the foot and ankle (foundation of the body) very unstable. PCOs apply vertical lift (support) right where this twist is, in the front of the foot.

An arch support does not put support where the twist is; it puts it further back in the foot, under the arch area where it is not as effective. Conventional orthotics also utilize the arch area of the orthotic as a fulcrum to influence foot and body functioning. Also, most conventional orthotics have control under the rearfoot (back of the foot) under the heel; again, neither of these areas, the heel or the arch, is where the problem really is and where the control needs to be.

The amount of vertical lift needed to control an excessive pronator is often rather substantial. Most conventional orthotics are made out of semi-rigid and rigid materials; such high vertical wedge requirements would force patients to slide off of these orthotics. They would become totally ineffective. However, PCOs are Class II mechanical levers, as compared to conventional orthotics, which are Class III mechanical levers. PCOs have a longer fulcrum arm and, therefore, can exert more force than conventional orthotics to combat and offset excessive pronation.

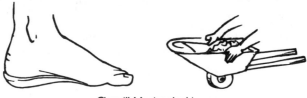

Class III Mechanical Lever

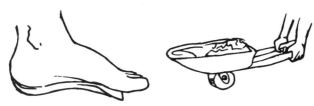

PCO Class II Mechanical Lever

The amount of vertical deficit is measured by a BioVector™, which is made out of the same materials that the PCO is. Thus, we are able to get a very precise measurement of the exact amount of vertical correction needed. With other orthotics, you are usually not able to quantify the amount of correction they are supposed to have in them. More importantly, PCOs allow the practitioner to verify the prescription by measuring them directly before being dispensed to the patients.

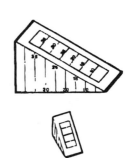

BioVector

Posture Control Orthotics and Shoes

Fitness shoes (walking, running, aerobic, cross-trainers, etc.) with removable inner soles are the best shoes to use with Posture Control Orthotics, especially during the break-in period.

BioVector Measuring Forefoot Varum

Whatever shoes you use should:

1. Be relatively light in weight.

2. Have a lacing system

3. Be fairly flexible where the toes bend.

4. Have heels that are broad and preferably no more than one inch high.

5. Have the heel's counter hold your foot firmly in place.

6. Have the orthotic fit all the way back in the heel against the inside bottom of the shoe.

7. Have the front portion wide and high enough in depth to allow the front of the foot and toes to move comfortably with the orthotic in the shoe.

8. Be made of a soft material to mold around the foot.

Posture Control Orthotics are usually not made to function in high-heeled shoes. They also may not fit in some more stylish flat dress shoes.

Case Histories

The following chapters deal with specific case histories concerning actual patients who have undergone Posture Control Orthotic Therapy for various types of painful postural conditions.

The length of time in therapy depended upon many variables but especially on degree of pronation, time of onset, duration and number(s) of symptoms, age and weight of patient.

5

Case History: Chronic Pains – Foot to Head

P atient was referred to my office by a physician, because of chronic pain syndromes, literally foot to head. She was in her early thirties and in good general health. Her problems actually started several years ago, due to an injury she sustained while working as a hospital nurse. She had been trying to lift a patient, fell, and injured herself. She has had trigger point injection therapy and ongoing physical therapy for quite a while, with moderate success. However, symptoms would eventually recur. She admitted to having the following complaints:

1. Recurrent headaches.

2. Neck and shoulder tension.

The above complaints related to a TMJ disorder for which she was receiving treatment from a dentist who specializes in this type of work.

3. Tingling down the right arm.

4. Pain in both hips.

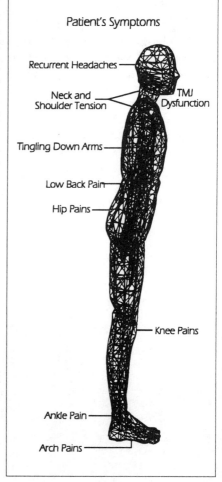

Patient's Symptoms

Recurrent Headaches

Neck and Shoulder Tension

TMJ Dysfunction

Tingling Down Arms

Low Back Pain

Hip Pains

Knee Pains

Ankle Pain

Arch Pains

5. Low back pain, especially on the right side.

6. Pain on the outside of the right knee, outside of the right ankle and on the bottoms on both arches.

Biomechanical evaluation revealed the following:

1. She had excessive pronation bilaterally.

2. Joint range of motion in both feet was relatively flexible.

3. Mild bunion joint formation right and left.

4. Adequate range of motion at the ankle joint.

5. Knock-kneed.

6. Swayback appearance, a forward protraction of the shoulders, and her head was thrust forward.

7. She seemed to function with a limb length discrepancy, with a premature heel lift right, suggesting a shorter right limb.

8. Excessive muscle tension throughout her body.

Biomechanical measurements revealed that she had asymmetrical excessive forefoot varum, measuring 0/18mm right and 0/15mm left foot. She was, therefore, calibrated for her first pair of orthotics posted at 0/5mm right and 0/4mm left. I elected to go ahead with a very conservative approach because of the chronicity and the multiplicity of the problems, as well as the severe muscle tension that she had.

The orthotics were dispensed several weeks later. She was given precise break-in instructions, both orally and written. I also suggested, since she was not able to work, that she should utilize good supportive fitness shoes all the time.

She was next seen several weeks later. As I had anticipated, because of her particular situation, she was having a hard time getting used to the orthotics. It had been three weeks since she had started using them, and she was barely able to wear them for two hours a day without being very sensitive in her feet and experiencing muscle spasms in the lower legs, right hip and groin areas. I watched her walk, I remeasured her biomechanically, reassessed the orthotics and did not see any contraindications to them or to the control on them. I suggested she try and bear with it until she got more used to them.

I next saw her one month later, and by then she was up to four hours a day. The devices were starting to feel more comfortable, and the muscle spasms were no longer present. She had no new complaints, but most of the old symptoms were still present, though some, from the foot up to the hip, were starting to decrease slightly.

She was next seen in my office about six weeks later. She had the following to report:

1. Headaches - gone.

2. TMJ pain - 80% better.

3. Shoulder pain, stiffness - decreased.

4. Tingling down the right arm - still present.

5. Left hip - almost no pain at all.

6. Right hip - getting better, not quite as painful.

7. Low back - better.

8. Right knee - better.

9. Right ankle pain - gone.

10. Plantar Fasciitis (arch pain in the feet) - gone.

Obviously, overall she was doing much better, and I suggested we did not have to see her again unless she stormed.

Approximately three weeks later the pain storm occurred. She started noticing some of her symptoms recurring. Therefore, some temporary materials were placed on the bottom of her orthotics, and she was calibrated for a second pair, posted at 0/8mm left and 0/9mm right.

Subsequently, she went through two more pairs of orthotics. Her last pair was posted at 0/20mm right and 0/19mm left.

After an appropriate break-in period, and checkup several months after that, she reported that all the symptoms from the foot to the hip were totally gone. She had mild discomfort in her low back after trying to do some fitness walking every other day. She also still had about 20% of the problems related to her TMJ dysfunction, i.e., the neck and shoulder stiffness. The headaches and right arm numbness, which had recurred, were gone. Obviously, she was very pleased overall.

She is anticipating going back to school and work eventually, for the first time in four years. She was advised, based on the measurements that I took, that unless she stormed, I would not have to see her again until a new pair of orthotics was indicated.

6

Case History:
Jaw Pain and Headaches

A 42-year-old female presented herself to the office with the chief complaint, "I've had a problem with my jaw all my life." She had worn braces on her teeth as a child, and was somewhat disappointed because the teeth were moving again. She also stated that her jaw hurt all the time, and she noted popping, clicking and grinding in her jaw, left side more than right. The problem seemed to be getting worse.

She also had another chief complaint involving a history of headaches that mainly occurred in the front of her head, behind the eyes. These sometimes would last for one or two weeks.

She also had a chronic back condition, with pain emanating from the mid and low back (sacroiliac joint area). This pain was especially noticeable whenever she got up after sitting for any period of time. She had been treated by a chiropractor and an osteopath.

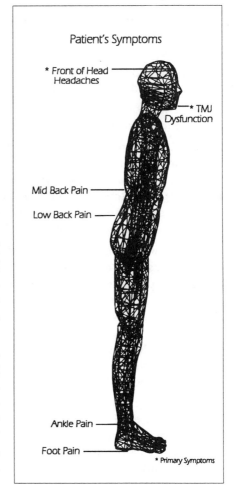

Patient's Symptoms

* Front of Head Headaches

* TMJ Dysfunction

Mid Back Pain

Low Back Pain

Ankle Pain

Foot Pain

* Primary Symptoms

She had another secondary complaint of left foot and ankle problems. She did not recollect any traumatic episode to either, and had no history of weakness or sprains there as a child. She had been diagnosed as having a bone spur in the left foot.

The pertinent physical findings were as follows:

1. The joint range of motions of the right foot were looser than the left foot.

2. No apparent leg length discrepancy was noted at this time; however, the patient had been receiving ongoing chiropractic and osteopathic care for pelvic instability.

3. The sternocleidomastoidis muscles on both sides of the neck were very tight.

4. The levator scapulae (neck) and the trapezius (shoulder blade area) muscles were very tight, right more than left.

5. The abductor muscles on the inside of the thigh and the hamstrings in the back of the thigh were very tight in both legs.

6. The hip flexors, the muscles that bend the hip, were tight, right side more than left.

7. Forefoot varum patterns were noted bilaterally, right measuring more forefoot varum than the left.

The overall conclusion was that the patient had excessive pronation due to an inordinate amount of forefoot varum, right pronating more than left. There was also a severe postural collapse with consequential abnormal muscle tension. Therefore, she had a contraction (tightening) in the muscle groups in the upper front of the body. She also had a lengthening (stretching) of the muscles in the back of the body.

Patient was put in her first pair of Posture Control Orthotics (PCOs) several weeks later, and had her first follow-up visit two weeks following. She had no problem with them for the first four days. Then she started getting some reactions. She had aching in her feet, ankles, and the back of her calves, as well as in her low back area. After a few days, this achiness went away. As far as her original complaints were concerned, there essentially was no change yet in any areas, except that the left ankle was a little better, and she felt more stable on her feet when she walked. She was rescheduled to be seen in three months.

On the next visit, she was doing a lot better. All symptoms, except for the jaw area, had receded appreciably. However, about ten days previous, her low and middle back areas started to bother her again. About seven days previous, she had started to have problems in her right shoulder, with some pain and clicking was associated with certain activities. This was a very old problem that she had forgotten about, and had not indicated on her initial visit.

The patient was reassessed biomechanically, and her vertical height measurements (forefoot varum measurements) had changed. This is consistent with pain storming. Therefore, temporary vertical lifts were added to her existing Posture Control Orthotics, and she immediately noticed that her mid-back symptoms were less irritating.

She was next seen in the office about four weeks later, when she stated that her low back ache was dramatically less, and the right shoulder pain completely gone. She did have some reactions to the temps (temporary vertical lifts) in her knees and her shins, indicating that she was somewhat sensitive to the changes in the tracking. She was then fitted for her second pair of PCOs. They were dispensed a month later.

In her follow-up visit for this pair, approximately one month later, she had been wearing them full time. They were still only semi-transparent, meaning that she still felt irritation from the front of the orthotics, in front of her foot and arch, after wearing them for more than eight hours. This is something that can sometimes occur and eventually does go away. She had had reactions to them in her left knee, a new symptom. This would indicate that her body was again sensitive to the changes in the tracking patterns that her PCOs were causing. Her left ankle was burning on the inside sporadically, also a new symptom. The shoulder blades in her upper back were very stiff and tight. However, overall, her right shoulder was still a lot better, with less popping and clicking during the same motions and activities that produced these previously. Her low back felt worse, both in intensity and frequency. On the other hand, she felt like she had much more energy, and said, "I feel taller, and straighter." She also felt more stable with these orthotics than in the first pair.

The patient was next seen approximately three months after her last visit. She had done fine during that time, stating that most of her symptoms had reduced, if not totally disappeared — including her headaches, jaw, ankle and back problems. However, approximately three weeks prior to the visit, she had felt she was going through another pain storm. Her left ankle and knee had started to ache again sporadically. She had noted a tightness in her neck, and she had begun to get headaches again, approximately three a week. Temporary vertical lift was again applied to the front of both of her orthotics. Immediately, walking with the temps on, she noticed less tension in her neck; this was corroborated by a physical examination.

She was seen again in a couple of weeks for a re-evaluation. By this time, the pain in her left ankle and knees was gone, the headaches almost gone, frequency had reduced from three times to no more than once per week. Her neck was better, looser. She did have some reactions to the orthotics, in terms of having some aching in her legs. She also stated that her low back had improved and the sciatica symptoms that had started to develop before this visit, in her left hip to knee, were better. She had had some problems with pain and numbness on the right side of her upper body and arm, but then had started to feel better.

Six months later, she came back to the office and stated that she had gotten much better with all of her symptoms, including her right arm.

The patient was seen periodically over the next year and received two additional pairs of orthotics. After her fifth pair, she came back stating, "These are really great." She had had some reactions getting used to them, mainly in the shoulder blade area, but that had not lasted long. "I feel more erect. I can't believe it — I haven't had any headaches for so long. I've forgotten about them. My mid back is fine," she said. Watching her walk, one could see that her shoulders were straighter, her posture better, the pelvic tilt had resolved, and she appeared to be within a couple of millimeters of vertical when she stood and walked. She had had no history of ankle problems or low back problems for over six months.

The patient then underwent one more pain storm, was measured and finally given her last pair of orthotics. This pair had 21 millimeters of forefoot varum in the right orthotic and 17 millimeters forefoot varum in the left orthotic.

Overall evaluation of this patient is as follows:

It is anticipated that she will not need to go through any more Posture Control Orthotic Stage Therapy, and the last pair of PCOs will only have to be changed every few years, due to the fatigue of the materials in the device.

What we have seen is an unwinding of the posture from foot to jaw. As we increase the vertical height, the symptoms start to resolve, usually from the ground, working up to the jaw. When a patient is experiencing a pain storm, then more vertical height is necessary. Then the patient will experience a period of feeling better, unless they storm again. If they experience another pain storm, the vertical height is increased again in order to get them asymptomatic. This is a fairly typical patient, demonstrating the use of incremental posting (vertical lifts) to attenuate and resolve postural pain issues.

Case History: Low Back Pain

A 31-year-old female was seen in my office because she had had chronic pain in the back for years. The diagnosis that she had been given by another doctor was sacroiliac joint dysfunction and muscle spasms in the low back. She used to be an avid fitness person, running and doing aerobics regularly. However, because of the low back problems, she had not been able to do any fitness activities for over two years. She was currently receiving physical therapy treatments once every two weeks, and had had conventional orthotics made approximately one year previously. The orthotics seemed to help her about 30%.

Biomechanical evaluation and gait analysis revealed:

1. Excessive pronation bilaterally.

2. Right foot pronates more than left foot.

3. Measured 17mm forefoot varum right, 14mm forefoot varum left.

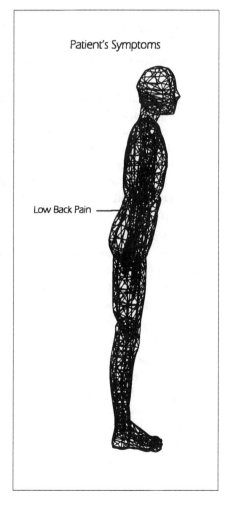

Patient's Symptoms

Low Back Pain

4. Excessive tightness in the muscle groups in the lower and upper back areas.

5. Knock-kneed, with a swayback appearance; shoulders protruded forward; head thrust forward also.

6. Left leg shorter than right.

7. Joint ranges of motions in the feet, ankles and knees were within normal limits; restriction in the low back area.

She was calibrated for her first pair of orthotics, which were posted at 0/9mm right and 0/8mm left foot.

The orthotics were dispensed a few weeks later, and a few weeks after that, she was again seen in the office. She had been able to wear them full time in about ten days after receiving them. They had been very comfortable, and there were no new symptoms or problems to report. She had felt more erect and more stable with the orthotics than without them. She still had not noticed any reduction of her back symptoms. However, they were not any worse. I suggested that she continue wearing the devices. I would not reassess her for approximately three months, unless the back symptoms increased or she experienced a pain storm.

A few months later, she complained that she thought she was storming. What had happened was that she started to feel better a few weeks previous, and she had been able to run a few laps around the track without any discomfort. By the end of the day, her back seemed to tire and bother her, but nothing like it used to. She had been able to increase the time between her visits to her physical therapist. However, two weeks prior to her visit to my office, she had noticed that the back felt more tired at the end of the day, and she assumed this could be a pain storm.

She was remeasured biomechanically, and indeed the numbers had increased. She now measured 21mm right and 17mm left. She was calibrated for her second pair of orthotics that were posted 13mm right, 11mm left. These orthotics were dispensed several weeks later.

She had no trouble breaking them in; she felt comfortable in them. The back symptoms started to recede again. She was contemplating getting back into regular athletic activities when I gave her the okay.

Since that time, she has had two more orthotic pair changes. Her last pair of orthotics, which was her fourth pair, was posted at 22mm right and 20½ mm left. Since then, she has felt good and has had minimal to no back pains. She has not seen her physical therapist in about four months, and is currently running about one mile every other day without any pain. I do not anticipate any other orthotic changes. When and if the current pair wears down, then a new pair, posted similarly to the last, would be made.

Case History: Chronic Knee Pains

D J.L., a 25-year-old male, 5 feet 10 inches, 150 pounds, had a chief complaint of a chronic, sharp-to-dull ache along the medial compartment (the inside of both knees), left more than right, for years. Symptoms increased with activity; however, sitting with knees bent produced stiffness. There was no history of any injury. X-rays were negative for boney involvement; however, some narrowing was noted along the inside aspect of the knee joint line, left more than right. Physical examination for ligament and other soft tissue injuries were negative for both knees.

Careful questioning divulged the following secondary symptoms in addition to the chronic knee problems:

1. Chronic fatigue in both feet at the end of the day.

2. Chronic ankle instability, tendency to turn his right ankle easily when playing basketball.

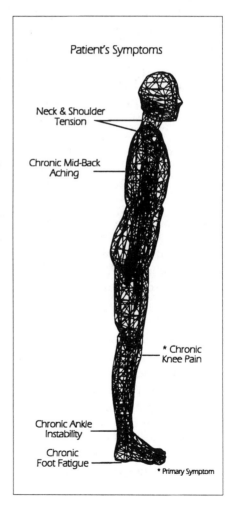

Patient's Symptoms

Neck & Shoulder Tension

Chronic Mid-Back Aching

* Chronic Knee Pain

Chronic Ankle Instability

Chronic Foot Fatigue

* Primary Symptom

3. Episodic clicking in his right hip, outside aspect.

4. Chronic mid-back aching, increasing with prolonged sitting or standing.

5. Chronic tightness in right shoulder and neck, increasing during the day

6. Had not been able to run comfortably for 10 years.

Examination: Pressure on the inside of the knee joint line elicited 1+ sensitivity right, and 3+ sensitivity left (on a scale 0 to 5, with 0 being least sensitive and 5 being very sensitive). Sensitivity was also noted on the tops of both legs, just below the inside of the knee joint. The tensor fasciae latae muscle ends in a connective tissue band called the illiotibial band, which itself ends on the upper portion of the outside of the lower leg, just below the knee. This illiotibial band was noted to be sensitive upon pressure to the right leg. There was also sensitivity noted on the back of the inside portion of the knee joint. This is an area where the muscles on the inside of the thigh, called the adductors, end. The sacroiliac joints in the back were extremely sensitive, 5+ left and 2+ right.

With the patient on his back, the left leg appeared ½ inch longer than the right leg. Lying on his stomach, both legs appeared to be the same length. The scapula levator and sternocleidomastoides muscles in the neck area were tight, right side over left side. The muscles that bend the hips (hip flexors) were extremely tight, left over right. The muscles in the back of the upper thigh (the hamstrings) were tight, 3+ for both right and left legs. In a standing position, with the knees bent, a knock-kneed (genu valgum) appearance and collapse of the inner-longitudinal arch was noted on both extremities.

Measurements: Forefoot varum 13 millimeters left, 17 millimeters right. This was measured standing on a BioVector, a biomechanical measuring device used to measure excessive amounts of pronation. Tibial varum, where the outside of the heel is on the ground, and the inside of the heel is off the ground a certain amount, of 4 millimeters bilaterally (using rearfoot wedges). There was adequate range of motion in the ankle joints, as well as other key joints in both feet.

Gait Evaluation (Visual Analysis): The heel bone (calcaneus) was excessively pronated at heel contact, right over left. The right foot was more turned out (abducted) than the left. Excessive pronation was noted upon walking, left over right. Knock-kneed (genu valgum) was noted, left over right. A pelvic tilt (hip tilt) was present, and he had a swayback. The right shoulder dropped during walking. The right arm swing was flimsy and weak. Both hands were in a pronated (turned outward) position. The patients drifted to his right side when his attention was diverted. The head was thrust forward and leaned toward the right side.

Treatment: **Day 1:** Postural Control Orthotics were fitted with a forefoot vertical lift, 5 millimeters left, 7 millimeters right. Patient stated, "My balance is off." Concomitantly, pressure awareness (not discomfort) was described along the inside margin of the end of the PCOs. A slow break-in period was stressed, with increase of wear time one hour per day as tolerance permitted.

Week Two: Mr. D.J.L. was able to wear the PCOs full time. Initial postural reactions: Increased aching along the inside joint line of the both knees. On Day 4, increased mid-back pain associated with standing or bending. On Day 7, increased fatigue in both legs and feet. However, all foot symptoms had dramatically improved, and he could stand longer before the mid-back began to ache.

Week Nine: The knee symptoms had dramatically improved. For the first time in five years, he was able to hike all day without debilitating knee pain; however, his knees were tired at the end of the hike. His mid-back was improved. He could sit and stand for longer periods of time before experiencing back discomfort. His feet continued to be asymptomatic. He felt his balance was improved and he was not drifting to the right as much as before. He felt as if he was standing straighter.

Week 23: Patient had begun "storming" approximately two weeks prior to this visit. Pain on the inside part of the left knee had recurred. Concurrently, his mid-back was aching, and his balance had deteriorated to the point where he was drifting to his right again. His feet continued to be asymptomatic. Front of the foot measurements were retaken.

Week 24: Subjective pain in the left knee was dramatically improved. Patient was measured for a second pair of PCOs.

Week 26: A second pair of PCOs was dispensed, with an increased vertical lift in the front of the orthotic 8mm left, 11mm right.

Week 32: Knees were continuing to improve. Patient was able to run three times per week, two miles per run, without significant knee pain. His mid-back no longer ached when he stood or bent, and was only mildly symptomatic when he sat more than two consecutive hours. His neck and right shoulder symptoms were abating. He has gone three or four days without any upper body stiffness. Once again, his balance was improving; he no longer drifted to the right.

Week 50: Stiffness in the right shoulder was recurring approximately one week prior to this visit. However, his knees and mid-back were no longer a problem. Foot measurements were retaken.

Week 51: Within 24 hours after temps had been applied, stiffness in the neck receded. The patient was remeasured for another pair of PCOs.

Week 53: The third set of PCOs were dispensed with a vertical lift of 12mm left, 15mm right. A 1mm lift was added to the back of the (rearfoot) left PCO. A 3mm lift in the back of the (rearfoot) was added to the right PCO.

Week 59: Patient was able to run 40 miles per week with no knee pain. All mid-back symptoms had subsided and, for the first time in his adult life, his neck was not tight, even under stress.

Week 83: Patient continued to do well. He was asymptomatic when he did not exceed structural limitations. Overall, the patient stated his foot was 100% improved, knees 75% improved, mid-back 80% improved, and neck 70% improved.

Special Note:

This patient was part of a study dealing with 128 people who had chronic knee pain. The study was conducted over a four-year period. All these patients had been treated prior to this study with various treatment modalities, including anti-inflammatory medication and aggressive physical therapy; some had had surgery. Results were disappointing. Pain was still present, and treatment had not met patient's expectations. All these patients had been professionally advised that nothing else could be done. Many were referred to Pain Management facilities to learn "body hardening" — how to cope with their pain and live with their disability.

See Appendix I, "Knee Study," for more information.

9

Foot Pains

C ase History A: Heel Pain

Mr. P.G., 52-year-old male, came into the office with severe pain in the bottom of the left heel. Biomechanical evaluation revealed that he had medium arch height when not on his feet. Arch height on weight-bearing was low. He had a flexible range of motion below the inside of the ankle joints and the first meta-tarso-phalangeal (behind the large toe) joints of both feet. The feet appeared to exhibit excessive pronation, looking at them from the back of the heels. He had a mild bunion deformity bilaterally. He had adequate range of motion at the ankle joint. He walked with his feet in a slightly out-toed position and his knees were knocked. He exhibited excessive asymmetrical forefoot varum, measuring 17mm forefoot right and 15mm forefoot left. He also exhibited some tension in the muscles in the back of the

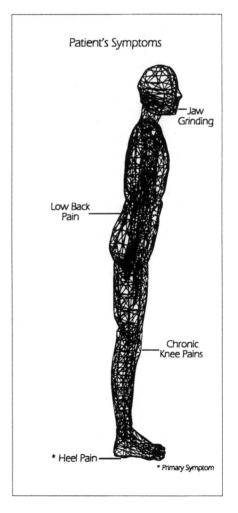

Patient's Symptoms

Jaw Grinding

Low Back Pain

Chronic Knee Pains

* Heel Pain

* Primary Symptom

body, and had marked trigger points, consistent with myofascial syndrome, in both calf muscles.

Other skeletal system symptoms included:

1. Jaw grinding, but no pain.
2. Low back pain; saw chiropractor regularly in the past, not as severe now.
3. Knee pains, occasionally severe over the last 10 years. Had X-rays done six years ago by an orthopedic doctor. Told there was a slight deterioration in both knees, but not to worry or do anything about it.

He was measured for a pair of Posture Control Orthotics, posted at 0mm rearfoot right and left, 6mm forefoot varum right, 5mm forefoot varum left. The orthotics were dispensed approximately three weeks later. He was given the orthotics with both oral and written instructions. He was seen about two weeks later, and still had problems with his left heel, his right knee, and some low back pains. By his next visit, some three weeks later, he was able to wear the orthotics all the time, after about a two-week break-in period. He had one new problem that developed in his right hip, lasted for several days and went away. His knees were still bothering him, especially the right, and the left heel was still sensitive, but was already 70% improved. Patient was to be seen in three months, unless he stormed or had any problems.

About one month after this visit, I received a call because the patient had sustained an injury to his right knee. This occurred in an accidental fall, and he sought orthopedic care because he could hardly walk. Both knees were X-rayed; he was told he had degenerative arthritis in them, and was given physical therapy and rest. It was then suggested to him that he probably would not be able get rid of the knee pain, and would have either to live with it or eventually have knee joint replacements, first the right, then the left. It was also recommended by the physical therapist and orthopedic surgeon that he should take the orthotics out, which he did.

After a few days, his feet started to bother him, especially the left heel. His body, in general, felt more fatigued, but the knees felt the same. The patient called me in distress, not knowing what to do. I offered to contact the orthopedic surgeon and physical therapist, and send them material about Posture Control Orthotic Therapy. I suggested that he start utilizing the orthotics again. When I spoke to the patient about two weeks later, he was wearing his orthotics and doing much better. The feet were feeling much better, the left heel was only slightly uncomfortable, and the knees were starting to feel better. His low back had not bothered him any more.

I saw Mr. P.G. about two months later. When he came in, his heels were feeling better, but the knees were starting to bother him again, and his low back felt a little tight, but not painful. He had been taking Motrin because of the knee problems, but had had to stop because of stomach trouble. I re-measured the patient biomechanically, and the measurements had changed significantly. He was measuring 23mm forefoot varum right and 21½mm forefoot varum left, as compared to 17mm right and 15mm left from the original visit. He was then calibrated for a new pair, measuring 12mm right and 11mm left. The original pair of orthotics was temped up, using 4mm of temp material right and left.

A few weeks later, the second pair of Posture Control Orthotics was dispensed. The heels were still doing great; the right knee was still bothering him, but it was no worse than the previous visit. Back was doing well.

Patient was seen again four weeks later for a check up on his second pair of orthotics. He had been doing very well with them, until he went from wearing them 8 hours per day to 14 to 16 hours in one day. After that, the right knee started to hurt a little. He said, "It felt like bone rubbing on bone." I reassessed the measurements on his orthotics and checked his shoes. I found him still to have posterior chain tension and suggested specific stretching exercises to be done two to three times daily. Also, I felt his shoes were too old. I suggested he get a new pair, that he use the orthotics 10 hours the following day, and then increase one hour per day until he was up to a full day's wear.

Patient was last seen two months later. He had no pain in his heels, knees or low back. He was able to wear the orthotics all the time, and had cut down on the stretching exercises to one time per day. He was ready to resume fitness walking, which he had not been able to do in one year. I went over a fitness walking program with him, and told him to call whenever he stormed or had any problems. The patient has not been seen in the office for over six months. He has not had a storm, and I anticipate that his excessive pronation may be controlled adequately with the second pair of orthotics.

Case History B: Bunion Joint Pain

Patient B.J., a 32-year-old female, came into the office with an extreme amount of pain in the bunion joints and the joints behind the second and third toes of both feet. She was an avid fitness person, who liked to run 25 to 40 miles per week. She had been doing this for several years with no real problems. Further questioning revealed no signs of overuse in her training. Her running shoes were new, with hardly any wear patterns noted.

Biomechanical assessment revealed that she was an excessive pronator. She measured 23mm of forefoot varum right, and 20mm forefoot varum left. Arch height was significantly reduced from sitting to standing; she had very flexible joint range of motions in her feet. She was severely everted on stance, right worse than left. She walked with a straight toe gait. Knees were knocked. She had signs of postural collapse, i.e., sway back appearance; head and shoulders were thrust forward.

X-rays revealed she had moderate hallux valgus (bunion deformities on both feet) and other signs consistent with excessive pronation.

Other secondary skeletal system symptoms included:

1. Neck and shoulder tension.

2. Occasional pulled muscle in her groin area, whenever she did any speed workouts, or when she would occasionally play softball.

3. Adductor (muscles on the inside of the thigh) strains in the past.

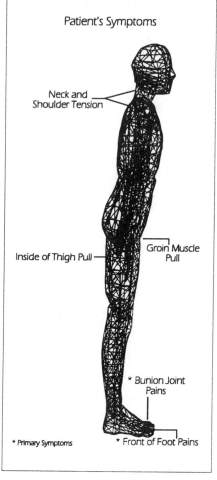

Patient's Symptoms

Neck and Shoulder Tension

Inside of Thigh Pull

Groin Muscle Pull

* Bunion Joint Pains

* Primary Symptoms

* Front of Foot Pains

She was calibrated for her first pair of Posture Control Orthotics, which were posted at 9mm forefoot varum right and 8mm forefoot varum left. Her first pair of Posture Control Orthotics were dispensed several weeks later. Appropriate oral and written instructions were given.

She was again seen in two weeks. By that time, she was able to wear the orthotics five to six hours per day. There were no new problems to report. Her chief complaint, which was her bunion joint pain, had receded significantly. But she was still having some pain in the joints behind the second and third toes; however, that was at least 50% reduced. She had no muscle pulls in her thighs. Neck and shoulder tension was still present.

When she was seen next in three months, she had been wearing Posture Control Orthotics all the time, except occasionally for work. She was running approximately five miles every other day, with a longer run on the weekend. She felt terrific. The neck and shoulder were a little better; no pain or problems with her groin. The adductor muscles did not feel tight; no injuries to them. Her bunion joints were fine, as long as she wore the orthotics. When she put on dress shoes and was unable to wear her orthotics, she had pain. When she went barefoot, the bunion joints still bothered her. The pain in the joints adjacent to the bunion joints was completely gone. Obviously, she was very satisfied.

Two months later, the patient was back in the office because of a pain storm. I re-measured her, and the measurements were somewhat higher. She measured 23mm forefoot varum right and 20mm forefoot varum left, as compared to 0/18½ right, 0/15½ left on the original visit. I temped up her first pair of orthotics, to 13mm right and 12mm left.

She was seen in the office three weeks later to pick up her second pair of Posture Control Orthotics. The stiffness and tightness in her neck and shoulders were getting progressively worse, but everything else was feeling much better. She initially felt uncomfortable with the second pair of orthotics, because they were longer and also had more control.

Two weeks later, she came in for her checkup; she was doing much better. All her symptoms had completely receded. She was very satisfied. She was able to run as far as she wanted, and was getting back into racing. I suggested that she be careful with her running program, and went over with her a gradual increase.

She was next seen three months later. About the orthotics, she said she "loved them!" She still measured 23mm forefoot varum right and 20mm forefoot varum left.

She came into the office six months later, still doing great. The orthotics were still at 13mm right and 12mm left. The measurements were the same as her last visit. She had no symptoms; her bunion joint pain was completely receded except when she had to occasionally wear dress shoes. She was completely satisfied. I suggested she be more judicious in the choice of dress shoes she wears and to consider getting a second pair of orthotics to fit specifically in her dress shoes. I also told her to call the office when and if she storms in the future.

10

Pediatric Problems: Four Case Histories

The following case histories include some types of pediatric biomechanical problems for which Posture Control Orthotic Therapy can be successfully used. It is interesting to note that, because of their youth, the patients' bodies have not been subjected to years of musculoskeletal abuse. Therefore, they usually respond more quickly than adults.

Case History A: Foot & Leg Pains Leading to Severe Physical and Psychological Problems

A seven-year-old female was brought into my office by her parents because she was having pain in her feet and legs after walking for short distances. She also complained of waking up in the mornings with stiffness in her hips and knees as well. She apparently had developed these problems approximately two years previously, when the parents noted she seemed to limp, especially on the left side.

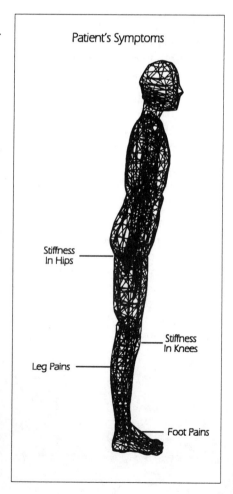

Patient's Symptoms

Stiffness In Hips

Stiffness In Knees

Leg Pains

Foot Pains

She also seemed to be very lethargic, i.e., would prefer to sit down, stay in bed and not stand up for any length of time. She also was somewhat withdrawn, and there was some concern about a psychological problem.

At the age of two, a hard object had fallen on her head, and she had suffered loss of consciousness. At that time a CAT SCAN was done, which was negative. She had recently been thoroughly assessed by a psychologist and an orthopedic surgeon. An MRI was done of the head; it had been negative. Blood tests were taken, and they were normal. The doctors couldn't find anything really wrong with her.

An extensive biomechanical evaluation and gait analysis was performed. Highlights of this examination revealed:

1. She exhibited a very low arch on sitting, and even lower when she stood up.

2. She had very loose and flexible joint range of motions in the feet.

3. She had adequate ankle range of motion.

4. Some limitation of motion on hip extension (straightening of the hip), left more limited than right.

5. Some weakness in the adductors (muscles on the inside of the thigh) and adductors (muscles on the outside of the thigh) of both legs.

6. Hip flexor muscles (muscles used to bend the hips) were weak.

7. Knee range of motion was within normal limits. No knee joint area abnormality noted.

8. The lower extremity reflexes were all normal.

9. Heel contact was severely everted bilaterally (sign of excessive pronation as seen from the back of the heels) in both feet.

10. Knee position was severely knock-kneed.

11. Gait pattern showed an out-toed gait.

12. On standing, there was a bulging of the talus bone and the navicular bone on the inside of the feet.

13. Severe, excessive pronation demonstrated during walking exam.

14. Her shoulders were protracted and the head thrust forward. The abdomen and buttocks were protruding excessively.

15. Biomechanical measurements of her feet showed she had excessive pronation due to excessive forefoot varum, measuring 0mm rearfoot (back of the foot) right and left, and 21mm forefoot (front of the foot) right and 22mm left foot.

My conclusions from the biomechanical exam was that she had excessive asymmetrical pronation, due to excessive forefoot varum measuring 0/21 millimeters right foot, and 0/22 millimeters left foot.

I discussed the concept of Postural Control Orthotic Therapy with her parents and we went ahead and calibrated her for her first pair of Posture Control Orthotics, that were going to be posted at 0/6 millimeters right foot, 0/6 millimeters left foot.

A few weeks later, the patient came into the office, and the first pair of Posture Control Orthotics was dispensed. Parents were given oral and written instructions. She was to be checked in approximately two to three weeks.

Approximately three weeks later, the patient came in for her first Posture Control Orthotic checkup. The parents could not believe the difference. She was still complaining of some problems with her hips after she sat for a while, but all other pains were completely gone. All the problems in her feet and knees had completely receded. The hip pain was better, but still evident after sitting. She was very stable on walking. She had had a little problem breaking the orthotics in initially, but was soon able to wear them all the time. She was able to stand, ambulate, and play for long periods of time, for the first time in several years, without problems or complaints. There was a dramatic improvement over her physical well-being and her mental outlook.

The parents were still concerned about the hips, and wanted to know what to do about it. I told them that they were certainly welcome to get a second opinion, but since their daughter had just started with PCO therapy, unless the symptoms increased, I would suggest, we give it a little more time. I anticipated rechecking her in about three to four months, unless the hips did not respond more or she experienced a pain storm.

Six months later, she was next seen in my office. Although she was completely asymptomatic, the father noted that her walking had started to become unstable again, and she tended to be a little clumsy. This apparently had been going on for several weeks.

New biomechanical measurements were taken, and indeed the numbers had changed significantly. She now measured 0/26 millimeters right foot and 0/29 millimeters left foot. Originally she was 0/21 millimeters right foot and 0/22 millimeters left foot. She was, therefore, calibrated for her second pair of Posture Control Orthotics, which were posted at 0/12 millimeters left foot, 0/11 millimeters right foot. The second pair was dispensed several weeks later.

On the checkup visit, she still had no symptoms, no problems. Stability in gait was apparent; no clumsiness.

Three months later, she was brought in by her parents for her checkup. She was doing fine, but had started to have some pain in the right hip. Upon further questioning, we found out that she had started to use a scooter about four weeks before, and this seemed to be the time the pain occurred. However, I watched her walk, re-evaluated her biomechanically, and again found out that the numbers had increased. The measurements were 0/28 millimeters right foot, 0/31 millimeters left foot. Therefore, we temporarily increased the control on the orthotics. She was then calibrated for her third pair of PCOs, which were posted at 0/21mm left and 0/20mm right. After a few weeks, the right hip symptom disappeared. All of her previous complaints were still receded. She looked very stable when she walked or ran.

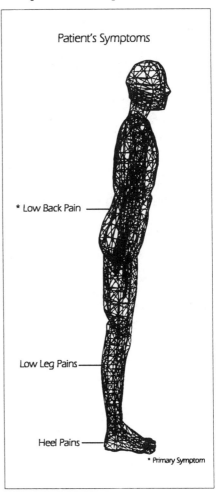

Patient's Symptoms

* Low Back Pain

Low Leg Pains

Heel Pains

* Primary Symptom

I told the parents that, based on my measurements, I thought that this could be her final pair of Posture Control Orthotics and that I would check her in approximately six months unless there was a pain storm. I anticipated these orthotics to last several years, until the materials weakened, or her foot size changed significantly.

Case History B: Back Pain

Patient M.P. was brought into the office because he had had a sore back for four months. The mother had a friend whom I had successfully treated for her back problems with Posture Control Orthotic Therapy.

M.P. was a twelve-year-old male in good general health. He was not allergic to or currently taking any medications. His low back had been bothering him for the last four months, especially after playing basketball. Because he had been going to basketball camp, he had had an ongoing pain all summer.

Past skeletal history included problems with pain in the front of his legs. His mother had been told these were "growing pains." He also had had pain in the bottom and back of his heels three years ago, called apophysitis (inflammation of the cartilage tissue in the back of the heels). There also seemed to be a history of back problems on the mother's side of the family.

Biomechanical evaluation was performed. The conclusion was that he had excessive asymmetrical pronation, which measured 0/19 millimeters right foot, and 0/17 millimeters left foot.

I explained the cause of the problem to his mother, and the relationship of his inefficient foot and leg functioning to the problems he had had with his heels, legs and low back area. He was calibrated for his first pair of Posture Control Orthotics, posted at 0/6 millimeters left foot and 0/7 millimeters right foot. He was also given recommendations for low back exercises to do daily. In addition, I suggested that he not go barefoot.

The first pair of orthotics was dispensed a few weeks later. The parents and patient were given explicit oral and written instructions on how to break them in.

Within two weeks, the patient was able to wear the orthotics all the time. He had had no problem with the break-in process. He had noticed that his back pain was no longer present when he was walking around or doing regular daily activities. He still had some discomfort when he was playing basketball for a long period of time. The feet, heels and legs had no problems. He had no other problems in his skeletal system.

Approximately three and one-half months later, he was seen again in the office. He had been having no problems with his back until approximately two weeks before the visit, mainly after athletic activity.

He was re-evaluated biomechanically, and he measured 0/25 millimeters right foot and 0/20½ millimeters left. I increased the orthotic forefoot control by using temps, so that he was now posted at 0/10 millimeters left foot and 0/11 millimeters right. He immediately felt relief, and was calibrated for his second pair of orthotics, posted 0/13 millimeters left, 0/14 millimeters right.

The second pair of orthotics was dispensed approximately two weeks later. After breaking them in, the patient had absolutely no pain again, was completely asymptomatic. He and his mother were both very satisfied. I told him to continue to do the stretching exercises every other day, instead of every day, and to continue to heed my advice about not going barefoot.

He was checked approximately four weeks later, and was still not having any problems. I told his mother that unless he outgrew the orthotics or had a pain storm, I would not have to see him again for approximately one year.

Case History C: Groin Pain

S.J., a seven-year-old female, was brought into the office by her mother because she noticed that S.J.'s feet were rolling in (collapsing) severely when she walked. This had become especially obvious during the last few years. In addition, the girl had started having some pain in the left groin a few months previous. She was examined by her pediatrician, who told the mother that there was nothing internally wrong with the groin area. He also felt that the problem might have to do with the way the feet rolled in. She was referred for consultation.

S.J. was in good general health, had no allergies, no childhood history of injury. The mother had worn special orthopedic shoes as a youngster. Upon furthering questioning, I discerned that S.J. had had problems with low back pain in the past, despite her young age, and had complained of some stiffness in the neck area from time to time.

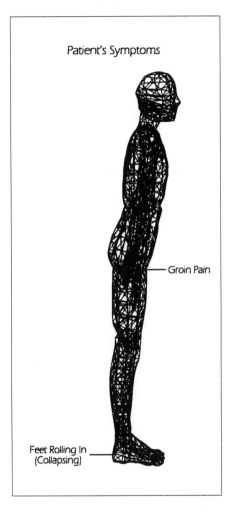

Patient's Symptoms

Groin Pain

Feet Rolling In (Collapsing)

Biomechanical assessment and gait evaluation was done, and the overall conclusion was that she exhibited excessive asymmetrical pronation which measured 33 millimeters right foot, and 26 millimeters left foot. The patient also had signs of severe postural collapse. The shoulders were definitely protracted, the head was thrust forward, the knees were knocked and the buttocks protruded excessively. She was calibrated for a pair of Posture Control Orthotics that would be posted at 0/12millimeters right foot, 0/10 millimeters left foot.

A few weeks later, the Posture Control Orthotics were dispensed to the patient. The mother was given oral and written instructions for breaking in the orthotics. In addition, she was instructed to get special shoes with a deep heel seat and a conventional type lacing system.

The patient was seen two weeks later for her first orthotic checkup. She was complaining that the devices were uncomfortable in the arches and that she had had knee pains, so she stopped wearing them. Adjustments were made to the orthotics so they would fit better in her shoes, and we suggested that she purchase a pair of thin insoles to wear over them for comfort. I also suggested that she break them in more slowly by starting to wear them 15 minutes the first day, 30 minutes the second day, then 60 minutes the third, and so on. In addition, I felt that the shoes she was using were too old and too small.

I told the mother that if the orthotics were still not comfortable in a few weeks, and/or the symptoms didn't go away, to please call and bring her in. Otherwise, I would see her in approximately three months.

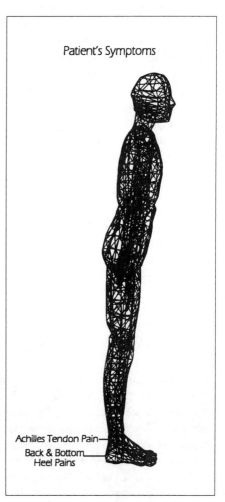

Patient's Symptoms

Achilles Tendon Pain—
Back & Bottom
Heel Pains

About three months later, S.J. was last seen in the office. The ankles and knee discomfort had receded. There was no groin pain at all. This had disappeared after she was able to wear the orthotics full time.

The patient has not had any further problems. She will be seen again if she storms, or if her foot and shoe size change significantly.

Case History D: Heel Pain

Patient J.R., a nine-year-old male, was brought into the office with severe heel pain in the back and bottom of the right heel for several weeks, the left heel for about one month. This problem had never occurred before. On squeezing the Achilles tendon, the patient also had exquisite pain in the back of both heels.

X-rays were taken, a biomechanical evaluation was done, and the resultant diagnosis was that he had apophysitis of both heels, an inflammation of the developmental cartilage in the back of the heels. He also had severe Achilles tendinitis in both heels and lower legs, due to excessive pronation.

Biomechanical evaluation revealed that he had asymmetrical excessive pronation, measuring 0/22 millimeters right foot, 0/20 millimeters left foot. He was calibrated for a pair of Posture Control Orthotics that would be posted at 0/12 millimeters right foot, 0/12 millimeters left foot.

His orthotics were dispensed a few weeks later, with oral and written instructions. In addition, he was given exercises to stretch the calf muscles of his legs daily, and instructed not to go barefoot unless he had to. The patient was scheduled to be next seen in a few weeks.

Because of severe winter weather, I did not see him again for about five weeks. Nevertheless, he was doing well. He had had no problems breaking in the orthotics; he was wearing them all the time. He had no pain in his heels or his Achilles tendons any more. He was able to participate in athletic activities again without problems.

I recommended that we check R.J. in approximately three months, unless he had a problem. At that time, he was still doing very well. He was now involved in running long distances, and the parents were ecstatic that he had no discomfort at all. I instructed the parents to contact me when and if he had a pain storm or a significant foot growth.

I did not see him for quite a while. Then they came into the office because the orthotics were irritating his feet because of foot growth. However, he had no pain. He was remeasured at 0/23 millimeters right foot, 0/21 millimeters left foot. He was calibrated for another pair of orthotics at the same time, with measurements of 0/13 millimeters right foot, 0/12 millimeters left foot.

The orthotics were dispensed a few weeks later. He was wearing them all the time after one week without problems; they felt comfortable, and there was no pain in his heels or Achilles tendons. He was instructed to be seen in the office if he had a pain storm, another significant growth spurt occurred, or in approximately one year, whichever came first.

Fitness / Sports Injuries: Four Case Histories

Case History A: Knee Pains

A thirty-year-old female came into the office complaining, "My knees hurt whenever I do any fitness walking, walking for a long time or even running for a short period of time." She had a history of the left knee dislocating at the age of sixteen, which was related to a sports activity at the time. She also found that the more active she was, the more the left kneecap seemed to feel unstable.

The right knee was also a problem for her, although she stated that the right kneecap was not as unstable as the left. The right knee problem had started in the second year of college, when she was involved in fencing.

The chief complaint she had, as mentioned above, was due to her knee problems. However, she did have other secondary complaints, which we are going to mention here for the sake of completion. She also had chronic headaches and upper back

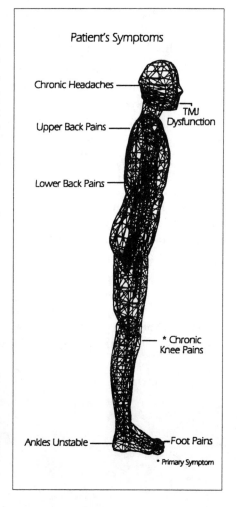

Patient's Symptoms

Chronic Headaches

TMJ Dysfunction

Upper Back Pains

Lower Back Pains

* Chronic Knee Pains

Ankles Unstable

Foot Pains

* Primary Symptom

problems that were related to a TMJ dysfunction for which she was receiving treatment from a dentist who specializes in this care. In addition, she had pain in her back and her ankles were unstable, left more than right. Finally, the arches of both feet were painful.

Biomechanical evaluation and gait analysis showed that she had excessive pronation, left appearing more pronated on stance than the right. She had very tight muscles when she walked. She had classic signs of postural collapse, which included excessive pronation, knock-kneed, sway back, shoulders protracted or hunched forward and the head thrust forward. In addition, the ankle joint range of motion was diminished, reflective of the tight muscles noted in the back of her body, left more than right. She seemed to have a definite functional leg length discrepancy, i.e., the left side functioned longer than the right, when walking. This was definitely related to one foot pronating more than the other, leading to an abnormal pelvic tilt. In addition, she had tight neck, shoulder and hip muscles. She had pain on palpation or pressure on both knees, left worse than right. She also had a grinding noise (crepitation) in the left knee.

The original measurements for forefoot varum showed her to have: asymmetrical excessive pronation, measuring 0mm rearfoot left and right, 20mm forefoot varum left and 24mm forefoot varum right. From these measurements, her first pair of orthotics, which were dispensed several weeks later, was posted at 8mm forefoot varum right and 6½mm forefoot varum left. No rearfoot posting was needed on the orthotics.

Patient was again seen approximately three weeks later. She was able to wear the orthotics all the time, after the first week comfortably. She did have some reactions to them. She noticed stiffness in the muscles in her thigh and her knees hurt her, but "in a different way." She still had her other symptoms, except she noticed that her low back was definitely improved.

Two months later, she was again reassessed in the office. Overall, her knees were definitely improved; the pain was much less frequent. She noted that her legs felt much straighter, i.e., she was well aware that she previously had a tendency to be knock-kneed, and the inside of her knees often touched or banged together. This apparently was much improved. All her other symptoms had regressed, except she still had problems related to her TMJ dysfunction in the neck and head area.

However, the week prior to coming into the office, she noticed that the symptoms that had previously receded were starting to come back. Therefore, I explained to her that this was what we call a pain storm. Temporary vertical posting of 4mm was added to both right and left orthotic. She felt immediate relief from some of her symptoms, especially in the knee and back area. Her second pair of orthotics was dispensed approximately three weeks later, and they were posted at 11mm right,

10mm left in the forefoot. After a normal break-in period, she was again assessed in the office. The knees were much better, especially the left knee. She was definitely standing more erect, her knees were straighter and the mechanics looked much more efficient when she was walking.

Three months later she came into the office and said, "I'm doing amazingly well." She had basically no symptoms. She and the physical therapist with whom she had been working had noticed that the muscles in her body had started to really relax and stay relaxed. Her joint range of motions, even in her upper body, was much more flexible than in the past. Even her dentist noticed that her jaw was moving a lot better than before. The left knee felt much more stable; her right knee was fine. She also felt that she was standing straighter and taller.

Apparently, a week or two before this visit, she had noticed that the progress she had made was again starting to recede, and she again was going through a pain storm. She was, therefore, temped up 4mm again on the forefoot of both orthotics, and she was calibrated for her third pair, which was posted at 17mm right, 15mm left.

Three months later, after a short break-in period, she was seen. Again, the results were excellent; her knees were not bothering her at all. She was able to do a good deal of fitness walking without any discomfort. Her other symptoms were also responding very positively, and she was told to call the office when and if she had another pain storm.

This occurred approximately three months later. Though she felt she was standing more erect, she noticed some of her symptoms coming back. Temps were given on this visit, and the symptoms started immediately to recede. Her fourth pair of orthotics was then dispensed, at 19mm forefoot left and 21mm forefoot right. After a short break-in period, she reported that all symptoms had completely receded again, with the exception of a mild discomfort related to the TMJ dysfunction problem in her jaw.

She was again checked three months later, and was still doing well. We recommended that she call the office when and if she experienced a pain storm. It also was suggested that she continue to do fitness walking, and, if she wanted to start running, to do so carefully and gradually. A running/training program was discussed. I also anticipated that this would be her last pair of orthotics.

Case History B: Chronic Achilles Tendinitis

Patient L.R. had been treated for over ten years for chronic Achilles tendinitis, especially in the left Achilles. The prime focus of the treatment had been conventional orthotics. He had had moderate success with these orthotics over the years, but his symptoms had been getting worse. No matter how he rested or stretched, he could not get rid of the pain, especially in the left Achilles area.

Upon questioning, he apparently had other symptoms that were consistent with a chronic pain patient due to excessive pronation.

1. Chronic headaches at the end of the day, which had been going on for years.

2. Neck and shoulder stiffness and pain for years.

3. Back and legs were sometimes achy and stiff by the end of the day.

A complete biomechanical and gait analysis was performed, and, essentially, the end result was that he had asymmetrical excessive pronation, which measured 0mm rearfoot varum right and left. He had 17mm forefoot varum right and 15mm forefoot varum left. He also had extremely tight muscles from foot to neck.

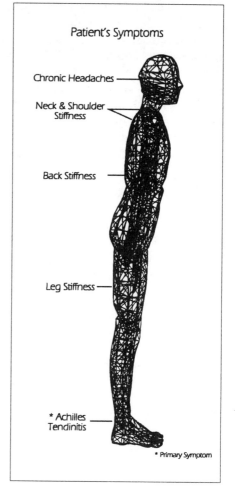

Patient's Symptoms

Chronic Headaches

Neck & Shoulder Stiffness

Back Stiffness

Leg Stiffness

* Achilles Tendinitis

* Primary Symptom

He was measured for his first pair of orthotics, which were calibrated at 0/12mm right and 0/11mm left. His orthotics were dispensed several weeks later with oral and written instructions. He was given an appointment for a check up visit several weeks later.

His Achilles tendinitis and pains in the back of the heels, left worse than right, were still about the same. Initially, he had worn the orthotics too long and had had some knee problems. But after cutting back the wear time and starting out again, these seemed to resolve. I suggested that he continue to utilize them all the time, and not get too frustrated, reminding him that the pain he had been having was ten-plus years old, and it would take time to respond to treatment. He was to be checked in three months, unless he had a pain storm.

He came back a week later, having tried to run in the orthotics. The left Achilles had hurt him quite a lot. After reassessing his situation, I decided that we would try to get more aggressive in our approach, and added two more millimeters of forefoot varum to his orthotics. He came into the office over two months later and had the following to report: The upper body symptoms were completely gone; the only thing that was still bothering him was the back of his left heel, mainly when he ran. When he did fitness walking for long periods of time, he had no problems. He had been able to run short distances for a while, but soon the pain in the left leg became too much for him to continue.

He was reassessed biomechanically, and his measurements had significantly changed. He now measured 23mm of forefoot varum right and 21mm forefoot varum left. We increased the temps on his current orthotics; 3mm forefoot posting to the right, and 2mm forefoot posting to the left. This gave him a total of 17mm right and 15mm left forefoot varum. In addition, he was calibrated for his second pair of orthotics, which were posted at 0/20mm right and 0/18mm left.

These orthotics were dispensed several weeks later. The patient went through the break-in period, and was seen several months later. He was doing great. He was able to walk without any pain in his heels. His upper body symptoms had completely receded. He started to work into a very gradual running program, and was now running 15 minutes every other day without any pain at all. I suggested that he call when and if he stormed. I have not seen the patient in over six months. We have spoken by telephone, and he is doing fine, still having no problems.

Case History C: Heel Spur Syndrome/Plantar Fasciitis

Patient G.S. is a 32-year-old female in good general health. She had come into the office because she had been having pain in the bottom of her right foot for approximately one year. She had been training for the San Francisco marathon and began having pain in the bottom of her right foot. She continued to train with the pain, and ran the marathon several months later. In order to help her get through the marathon, she was taking anti-inflammatory medication prescribed by another doctor. The pain kept bothering her, and she finally had to stop doing any running at all several weeks before visiting my office.

She stands on her feet all day at work and, for the last several months, had noticed that she had problems at the end of the day. When she was young, she had had problems with her right hip, which she was told became inflamed whenever she did any aggressive fitness activities, such as playing racquet ball. When she had stopped those types of sports and started to do running only, the right hip problem receded.

She usually prefers to run six to eight miles, five days per week, and wears relatively new running shoes, with no unusual sole wear. She said she tends to wear the front of the outsole of the shoe out, more than most people. She also works out with weights for her upper body four days per week.

Biomechanical evaluation and gait analysis revealed that she had excessive asymmetrical pronation that measured 0/25mm right and 0/21mm left foot. She has a partially compensated equinus when she walks. This means she comes off her heels too quickly, left worse than right, when she walks, and this is reflective of very tight muscles in the back of the body. In her case, after assessment, I believed the problem came from very tight upper and lower back muscles. She also had a tendency to function with a shorter left leg, due to the asymmetrical excessive pronation. X-rays showed that she had a calcaneal, or heel spur, on the bottom of the heel bone in her right foot.

Therefore, my diagnosis was that she had calcaneal heel spur syndrome and plantar fasciitis, i.e., inflammation of the plantar fascia (the ligament in the bottom of the arch) of the right foot. This was due to the asymmetrical excessive pronation, right worse than left.

Patient's Symptoms

Heel Pain - Plantar Fasciitis

She was calibrated for a pair of Posture Control Orthotics that were posted at 0/10mm right and 0/8½mm left. The orthotics were dispensed several weeks later, with oral and written instructions about how to break them in. We also discussed how to get back into a consistent running program gradually.

Because of bad weather, she was not able to get into the office as scheduled, and I did not see her for almost five weeks. By that time, she had been running inconsistently, due to the weather. The orthotics were very comfortable; she had been able to wear them all day. She had no pains when walking. When she ran, she still had some discomfort in the right heel and arch, but it was much better than before.

She was again seen three months later. At that time, she had no pain in the right heel, no pain in the right arch, and was running four miles every other day. She also contemplated starting to train seriously for an upcoming marathon.

I suggested that this pair of orthotics may be all that is necessary to control her problem, and that she was to call if and when she had a pain storm. I will reassess her in approximately one year.

Case History D: Shin Splints

Patient C.D., a 49-year-old female in good general health, came into the office because she has had a problem for three years with shin splints in both legs. The right was worse than the left. She apparently was running about thirty minutes every other day. On the days she didn't run, she cycled about forty-five minutes to one hour, and occasionally would swim for one hour on the weekends.

On the days that she did run, the legs, especially the right, seemed to bother her even when she walked, until the middle of the next day. She had new running shoes with no excessive wear patterns noted.

She had had a history of back problems, having undergone surgery ten years ago, and still had chronic low back pain. In addition, her legs fatigued rather easily, especially by the end of the day.

She also had a history of stress fractures in both lower legs

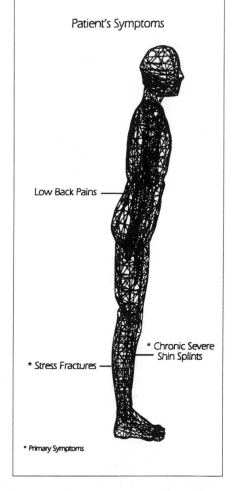

Patient's Symptoms

Low Back Pains

* Chronic Severe Shin Splints

* Stress Fractures

* Primary Symptoms

in the past, and at one time had had to take six months off in order to allow the fractures to heal. Nevertheless, when she started back to regular fitness activities, the problems continued. She also had to stand a lot at her job, which contributed to part of her problem. She had a history of aggressive, long-term physical therapy for her lower legs.

Biomechanical assessment and gait analysis was done. Overall conclusion was that she had asymmetrical excessive pronation measuring 0/23mm left foot and 0/25mm right foot. She also had excessive muscle tightness in the back of her body. She had marked trigger points, i.e., sensitive areas, in several muscles in the lower legs, especially the ones on the outside and inside of the lower legs.

She was calibrated for a pair of orthotics that were posted at 0/10mm left, 0/10mm right. They were dispensed approximately two weeks later. Even though she was again participating in fitness activities, I suggested that she not use the orthotics while doing these until I checked her again.

Three weeks later, she was seen in my office again. The legs felt somewhat better. She was still doing her fitness activities, and was not utilizing the orthotics for those yet, based on my instructions. She was having a little problem with the comfort in the front of the left orthotic and a minor adjustment had to be made on it. We discussed gradually breaking in the orthotics for her fitness activities.

She came into the office approximately two months later. Her legs were doing much better; she was up to running twenty-five minutes every other day, without any pain in the left leg and with only minor pain in the right. She was able to do her cycling without any problems. She was still on her feet all day at work, with no leg fatigue.

Unfortunately, she did sustain an injury to her back by lifting something incorrectly. She had had a minor setback, so we could not assess how the orthotics were doing for her chronic back pain at this time.

She was again seen three months later. The shin splints were fine; the low back was doing much better. She did not need another pair of orthotics at that time. I advised her that she may not need another pair, and to call me if she stormed.

This patient has had a tendency to overtrain and sustain periodic overuse injuries. I explained to her that if she did have a problem in the future, we would be able to know for sure whether it was overtraining or need for more control (vertical lift) on her orthotics.

When and if this injury did occur, I would reassess her biomechanically again, in addition to taking a running/training history. If the forefoot varum measurements had substantially increased, then more control on the orthotics would be indicated. My impression would be injury/pain due to a pain storm. If the numbers were the same or very close to where they were in the past, the problem would be due to overuse, improper training habits or excessive shoe wear. No change on the orthotics would be indicated. A review of her training program would be indicated.

12

Self-Examination And Self History

(How To Examine Yourself)

M ost people never put their assortment of pains together. However, headaches, joint stiffness, back pain and others — upon proper questioning — can reveal a pattern. That pattern often reveals a history of recurrent musculoskeletal problems which often seem to involve more pain, longer disability, and longer recovery periods as the years go by.

Many of us take it for granted that as we age, we will have some type(s) of postural pain(s), that we will be bent over and have stiff, painful joints. Believe it or not, this does not necessarily have to be the case. Posture Control Orthotic Therapy can often help correct poor posture and reverse the negative physical affects of the ensuing postural collapse.

The purpose of this chapter is to lead you through a self-assessment. Through your answers, you will know if you have suffered pain because of musculoskeletal reasons.

The second part of this chapter leads you through a physical self-examination in order to determine if you have inefficient foot and leg functioning due to excessive pronation. If you do, then Posture Control Orthotic Therapy could be beneficial for you.

Ask yourself the following questions:

1. How would you rate your general health? Good, fair, poor. People who are in poor health, who suffer from chronic infections or diseases, have a more difficult time coping with and recovering from recurrent chronic pain syndromes.

2. Past medical history. Have you had a history of hyperthyroidism, gout, hypoglycemia, anemia? These conditions can often lead to or exacerbate musculoskeletal pains.

3. Has anyone in the family had chronic postural pains in the past? Who, and what problems did they have?

4. Did you have any childhood history of orthopedic care for foot, leg or low back problem(s), or postural problem(s)?

5. Have you ever experienced any trauma, such as a car accident, falling off a ladder, athletic injuries?

6. If you do have postural pain(s), what would you consider is your primary problem(s)?

7. What have you done for your problem(s)?

8. Have you sought professional care? What was it? Neurologist, physical medicine, rehabilitation physician, chronic pain physician, orthopedic, osteopathic, counseling, chiropractic, orthopedic dentistry, physical therapist, massage therapist, podiatrist?

9. What treatment was rendered? Physical therapy, trigger point therapy, oral medications, anti-inflammatories, painkillers, bed rest, traction, surgery, acupuncture, some form of massage therapy?

10. Assess the different parts of your body, starting from the head down. If you've had any other problems, ask yourself: How long has the problem been there? Have you sought professional care? What was the diagnosis and treatment?

    a. Have you had recurrent chronic headaches?

    b. Any problem with your jaw/TMJ/clicking/pain?

    c. Any chronic neck or shoulder pain, stiffness, tension?

    d. Any pain or numbness, tingling, burning going down your arms, elbows, wrists, hands?

    e. Any problems in your chest, or upper back area between the shoulder blades?

    f. Any problems in your lower back?

    g. Hips?

    h. Knees?

    i. Fatigue, muscle spasms or muscle cramping in the upper or lower legs?

    j. Ankle pain or weakness?

    k. Heel and arch pains?

    l. Chronic foot problems?

    m. Do you have problems sitting still for long periods of time?

Physical Evaluation

Postural pains foot to jaw and chronic pain syndromes are often associated with abnormal postural mechanics. The main culprit is often excessive pronation of the feet. The following is a self-assessment guide to enable you to ascertain whether you have normal or abnormal body postural mechanics. This is best done by standing still and having someone else observe you from front, back and side.

Front view:

1. Place your feet and legs together; compare with the figures below.

2. Feet and legs should be straight ahead, with legs straight, and the knees having a slight distance between them, and over the center of the feet.

3. Do your knees touch (knock-kneed)?

4. Is there any space between your ankles?

5. Are your ankles together or touching?

6. Do you have two to three inches of space between the knees (bowlegged)?

7. Do your feet and toes tend to turn inward (pigeon-toed)?

8. Do your feet and toes tend to turn outward (walk like a duck)?

9. Are your kneecaps level with each other, or is one higher and one lower?

10. Does one arch appear to be lower and the other higher?

11. Does one shoulder seem to drop lower than the other?

12. Does one arm appear lower than the other?

13. Does one hip appear to be lower or higher than the other? This could indicate that you are functioning with one leg shorter than another. This is usually due to

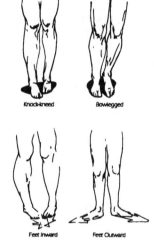

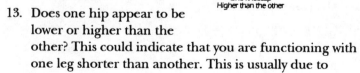

asymmetrical excessive pronation. This means that if one foot and leg pronates more than the other, it may function as a longer leg because it usually will be lower to the ground.

Side view:

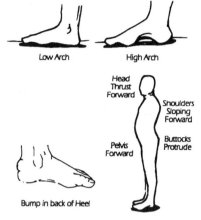

14. Do your arches appear to be equal in height? If so, would you classify your arches to be low, medium or high?

15. Do you have a bump protruding from the back of either heel?

16. Do your buttocks stick out?

17. Is your pelvis thrust forward, i.e., does your stomach protrude?

18. Are your shoulders sloping forward; are you round-shouldered?

19. Is your head thrust forward?

Along with excessive foot pronation, these are classic signs of postural collapse.

Back view:

20. Looking at the Achilles tendons in the back of your legs, does one or both appear to be curved outward somewhat, or are they relatively straight?

21. Check your legs again. Do they have the appearance of being bowed or knock-kneed?

22. Does one hip look higher or lower?

23. Does one hand hang lower than the other?

24. Does one shoulder appear to be higher or lower?

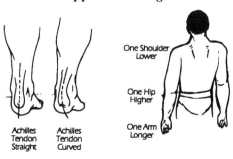

Now still checking from the back, bend your knees forward (hold on to a wall in front of you, so you don't fall) and have your examiner look to see if your foot arches collapse or flatten out more. Check to see if your ankles bulge or roll in more. Does the line in the back of the leg and Achilles tendon area curve more than it did? Do your knees tend to come closer together? These are all signs of excessive pronation, which can lead to postural collapse.

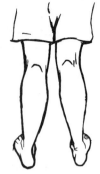

Ankles bulging inward
With knees bent forward

If your self-evaluation reveals an abnormal foot and leg structure, this can lead to inefficient foot and leg functioning and various postural pains foot to jaw.

Many people who have excessive pronation suffer from postural pains foot to jaw and chronic pain syndromes. However, the body tries to compensate for its weaknesses whenever it can. Some of us exhibit the classical postural collapse model, and others exhibit only some of this on initial examination due to the compensation.

You do not have to have all the postural signs associated with postural collapse to suffer from postural problems foot to jaw.

13

How To Choose Shoes

B esides fashion considerations, shoes essentially are used to protect our feet from the surfaces we walk on and the different climate conditions that our feet encounter, to help absorb shock and support us during our daily activities. They are the main environment in which our feet function. Since we wear shoes most of the time, we must be aware of the fact that they can have a profound effect on our bodies.

It is important to realize that shoes can have an impact both positive and negative on your postural pains. The following information should be used to help you choose the appropriate shoes to wear. There are four important points to consider about shoe wear:

1. Shoes must fit properly.

2. Worn down and/or old shoes can hurt you and should be replaced immediately.

3. Specific types of shoes should be utilized for different types of activities.

4. If you have musculoskeletal problems related to body mechanics, the choice of the shoes you wear can either help you or be detrimental to your ability to control or overcome your problems.

Fitting Process

Try on both right and left shoes. Have the shoes fitted while you are standing up. There has to be a fairly close resemblance between your foot's shape and the shoes. If not, you will not have a good fit and will not be comfortable using the shoes. You should not have to force a shoe on. No pinching or squeezing should be needed. If this is the case, these shoes are not the correct size for you; go up to the next size. The shoes should feel quite comfortable right away. They shouldn't have to be broken in, so to speak, for comfort's sake.

Go through the entire fitting process as described in detail below, first without your orthotics and then with them in the shoes, to see if the fit is good for you or not. Repeat the entire process for all the shoes you are interested in.

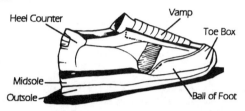

When you try on the shoes, make sure the heel of your foot is back against the inside of the heel counter of your shoe. You may have to gently tap the back of the shoe to get the heel of the foot in place.

Be sure there is one-half inch difference (usually a thumbnail's width) between your longest toe and the end of the shoe. Wiggle your toes around while you are doing this test, to see which one functions the longest when you stand, and also where it hits in the shoe. It is not uncommon to have the second toe, or even the third toe, be the longest.

The toes should fit in the toe box area at the front of the shoes with enough room to allow free movement of all the toes without pressure on the ends, tops or in between them.

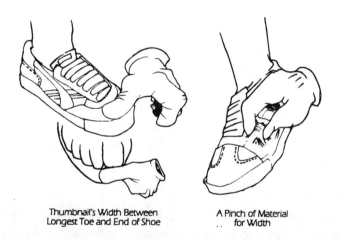

Thumbnail's Width Between
Longest Toe and End of Shoe

A Pinch of Material
for Width

The ball of the foot should be located at the widest part of the shoe. There should be a pinch of material available (while standing) in the ball area of the shoe for a proper width fit.

The heel counter should fit closely, but not too snugly either. Your heel should not be able to move or come out of the heel counter when stepping in place or walking forward. There should be only a slight, almost unnoticeable, slippage or movement of the heel in the shoe.

If possible, try to find a non-carpeted area of the store to use when being fitted and trying out your new shoes. You cannot tell much about cushioning, support, or the true feel of the shoe when on a carpeted area. Just putting shoes on and not really walking or mimicking your fitness activity in them may be deceiving. The actual action and motions your feet will go through in the shoes can affect their comfort, and, actually, the way the shoe fits. A shoe itself will change in length when you go from just standing in it, as compared to flexing it. When it is bent, the shoe actually shortens itself, and, if not fit properly, your toes will not have enough room at the end of the shoe. You may thus have to opt for a longer shoe size.

Worn Down and/or Old Shoes

A Posture Control Orthotic cannot support the body correctly in a worn down shoe. Excessive pronators generate a disproportionate amount of pounds per square inch throughout different parts of the shoe. In time, this leads to an uneven wear pattern, and the orthotic cannot support the body correctly. These people also wear the outside of their heels down excessively. When the outside is worn down significantly, the effects of the orthotics are obviously compromised, and they may become uncomfortable. Therefore, when the outside of the back of the heel or the sole of your shoe gets worn down between an eighth to a fourth of an inch at the most, they should be resoled or replaced.

Old vs. New

Very often, people will have fitness-type shoes that do not wear excessively in the heels, especially after getting Posture Control Orthotics. People may often have pain storms, come into the health professional's office and be re-evaluated, and the biomechanical measurements do not suggest that this is an actual pain storm. What is probably happening is that the midsole, which is the material between the insole and the outsole of the shoe, is worn down. This is responsible for shock absorption, and when this wears down or breaks down, both the orthotic and the foot tend to sit pronated on the inside of the shoe. This phenomenon, which we term the quicksand effect, can occur within months in certain shoes.

The general rule of thumb for the different types of fitness shoes midsole wear is as follows:

Aerobic – 100 hours

Cross Training – 150 hours

Running – 400 to 800 miles

Walking – 1000 miles

There is no simple timetable to go by with tennis and racquet court shoes. The best way to tell if these shoes are worn too much is when the front of the shoes can be easily bent and twisted from side to side. You will also notice more shock and stress in your lower legs.

Specific Types of Shoes Should Be Utilized For Different Types of Activities

Different fitness/sports activities have different requirements of your feet and your body. If you are going to be involved in a fitness activity fairly seriously, it behooves you to get the appropriate fitness shoe for that activity. For example, you would not want to do aerobic dancing in a running or walking shoe, because aerobic dancing requires side-to-side motion and running or walking is a straight forward motion. Trying to use a walking or running shoe for aerobic activities will break down the shoe quickly, and can lead to injury.

Different occupations have special shoe needs. If you are on your feet all day, and are required to do a lot of physical labor, you should purchase shoes with this in mind. Some work environments can lead to foot injury, and require special protective measures built into the shoes.

High-Heeled Shoes

In general, high-heeled shoes are really not good for anyone's feet. This is especially true if you are suffering from postural pains foot to jaw. However, if they can not be avoided in your life, you should try to wear as low heels as possible, and never get above two-inch heels. You should also attempt to wear flats as much as possible. Try switching heel heights every day —for example, a flat one day, a one-inch heel height another, then one and one-half inch heels.

The foot structure is designed to bear weight on specific parts of the foot, at specific times, during walking. High heels change the normal pressure distribution by pushing the foot forward. The higher the heel, the more pressure is transferred to the front of the foot. Though they

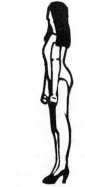

High-Heeled Shoes
And Postural Changes

may not cause foot problems themselves, they can certainly accentuate existing ones.

They can also foster poor postural alignment and, therefore, aggravate postural pains foot to jaw. They push your pelvis forward, your buttocks and shoulders backwards. This leads to a sway back posture, which can put a good deal of stress on your back. The muscles in your lower extremities become strained and fatigued. The back of the foot is positioned upward, and the front of the foot lower. This tends to shorten the calf muscles (muscles in the back of the leg), and strains the muscles in the front of the legs. This can lead to chronic postural pains.

Musculoskeletal Problems and Shoes

Comfortable feet are essential for correct posture when walking. Many aches and pains are caused by improperly fitted shoes or those with little or no support. Shoes that tie provide support and space for the foot, and are recommended when wearing shoes for long periods of time. Avoid slip-on shoes and those with wedge-type heels or thin soles, since they do not absorb the impact of walking, but put the stress on your body and its joints.

Shoes without laces, such as loafers and pumps, are generally fit short to avoid heel slippage. Such cramping can be detrimental, even though a person states the shoe fits and is comfortable.

Posture Control Orthotics and Shoes

More often than not, when problems are encountered using orthotics, solutions are found in the types of shoes they are worn in.

The best shoes to use are those with leather soles and rubber heels that do not compress, and thus provide an excellent platform for the orthotics. They should also be relatively light in weight, have a lacing system, and be fairly flexible where the toes bend.

The heel should be broad, and preferably no more than one inch high. The heel counter must hold your foot firmly in place. The orthotic should fit all the way back in the heel and be flat against the inside bottom of the shoe.

The front portion must be wide and high enough in depth to allow the front of the foot and toes to move comfortably with the orthotic in the shoe. Ideally, it should be made of a soft material to mold around the foot.

Athletic/fitness shoes, such as walking, running, and aerobic shoes, are usually very accommodating to Posture Control Orthotics. As mentioned before, when purchasing fitness shoes, the ones with removable insoles are more highly recommended.

No matter what type of shoes you use for your orthotics, the straighter the outsole is (the bottom of the shoe), the better off you will be. Turn your shoes upside down. You can either draw or make an imaginary line through the center of the bottom of the outsole. If there are almost equal amounts of material on either side of your center line, this is considered a straight-lasted shoe, and is excellent for people who are excessive pronators and wear orthotics. Most everyday shoes have a straight-last appearance.

The majority of fitness shoes are not made with a pure, straight-lasted outsole. They are usually made with a slightly curved last. Some are made with a more obvious curved-lasted appearance. This would have a lot more material under the outsole of the shoe, under the front inside of the foot, and not as much in the arch area. These are called semi-curved- or curved-lasted, depending upon the severity of the curve.

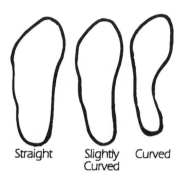

Straight   Slightly   Curved
                Curved

Posture Control Orthotics can usually be used effectively with straight- and slightly curved-lasted fitness shoes. However, the more severely curved-lasted styles are not as conducive to orthotics, and should be avoided.

Posture Control Orthotics are not made to function in high-heeled shoes. They also may not fit in some more stylish flat dress shoes. If this is the case, then a slimmer, modified type of PCOs is available and can fit into these types of shoes. This goes for both men's and women's shoe styles.

No matter what type of everyday shoes you wear, those made out of synthetic materials, such as patent leather, plastics and reptile skins, do not breath well, and often cause feet to get hot and sweaty.

Finally, remember always to take your Posture Control Orthotics and whatever number(s) and style(s) of socks you wear with you whenever you purchase new shoes.

14

Evaluating Your Nutrition and Weight

I t is well known that good nutrition plays an important role in our general health and well-being. As well, poor nutritional habits and inadequacies can impede and/or slow down one's ability to overcome postural pain/chronic pain syndromes foot to jaw.

Certain vitamins and minerals in adequate amounts, and in greater amounts during acute flare-ups, are helpful in promoting healing from these postural problems. These would include: Vitamins B1 (thiamin), B2 (riboflavin), B6 (pyridoxine), B12 (cobalamin); Vitamin C (ascorbic acid) and folic acid (folacin). In addition, you should ingest appropriate amounts of calcium, magnesium, potassium and iron.

You should take one Vitamin B Complex tablet daily after breakfast; one thousand milligrams of Vitamin C (time-release tablet) should be taken after breakfast and another one after dinner. If you smoke, you should double the dose per day of vitamin C.

Appropriate amounts of folic acid can be ingested through eating green leafy vegetables, organ meats and various milk products.

There are many books and sources of information available concerning foods that provide these vitamins and minerals and how much you need daily. I recommend that you go to your library or a book store, or consult your physician or health care professional to get more information about this. Nevertheless, the following healthful foods, if ingested in the proper portions, should fulfill most of your dietary needs: green leafy vegetables, various types of seafood including shellfish, poultry, lean meats, whole grain, whole grain cereals, nuts, citrus/dry fruits, various types of beans, lentils, potatoes, tomatoes, brewer's yeast, tofu, various dairy products, yogurt, cheeses.

The Weight Factor

Excessive weight is very unhealthy in general, and puts a lot of stress on the skeletal system structures, i.e., feet, legs, back, and neck.

If you suffer from recurrent postural pain/chronic pain syndromes foot to jaw, and already have a problem with inefficient foot and leg structure, i.e., excessive pronation, then your body is in a state of progressive postural collapse. Obviously, if you add unnecessary weight, this will only increase the tendency towards postural collapse, and perpetuate and exacerbate it. It could also interfere with your ability to overcome your problem(s). Hence, it is important that you consider losing weight.

Being overweight means that you weigh more than the average person of the same sex, age, and height. While some people are obese because of physical disorders, usually glandular in nature, most causes of obesity are due to poor eating habits, too much eating, or a combination of both.

There are limitless numbers of books and other sources of information concerning diet and weight loss programs. However, there is really no magic to it. What you need to do is use more calories per day than you take in. This is usually best accomplished by eating less food, and avoiding foods high in sodium, fat content and sugar. Participating in some form of fitness program will help not only reduce weight, but will firm up your muscles also.

Quick weight loss programs and fad diets are not only unhealthy, but in most cases have no lasting effects. It is just like treating a chronic pain syndrome patient's symptoms from time to time and not really dealing with the cause of the problem. Crash diets are usually a temporary fix and unsafe for your general health. They also never deal with the basic cause of your problem, which usually requires a general lifestyle change. This means eating less, eating more nutritionally, getting regular exercise, and, in some cases, getting professional counseling.

Before undertaking any radical dietary changes, I would suggest you consult your family physician or internist, especially if you have had any underlying physical problems such as diabetes or hypoglycemia.

Accomplishing this weight loss, through a permanent lifestyle change, will have a very positive affect on helping you overcome and control your postural pain/chronic pain syndromes foot to jaw.

General Health Considerations

While on the topic of the body's general health, there are certain physical conditions that can perpetuate chronic pain syndromes, and which need to be controlled through a health professional in order to fully overcome your problem. Some of the more common conditions are hyperthyroidism, hypoglycemia, anemia, diabetes, and chronic infectious diseases. In addition, people who have certain types of allergies and insomnia also find it more difficult to overcome these painful conditions, without appropriate care.

15

Position Is Everything – Sitting, Standing, Sleeping, Sex, Etc.

As we have seen, excessive pronation and postural collapse often lead to recurrent postural pain/chronic pain syndromes foot to jaw. Once they have compensated for the body's foundational inefficiency by utilizing Posture Control Orthotic therapy, most people start feeling better. Unfortunately, there are other factors that contribute to or perpetuate these painful condition(s). This chapter deals with some of these important perpetuating factors, how to recognize them and compensate for them.

Just as those people who have had success in losing weight and keeping it off are usually not those who go on crash diets, but who actually go through a lifestyle change, those who suffer from recurrent postural pains should change certain habits. These include how you sit, sleep, stand, get dressed, sit in your car, have sex, and so on. Essentially, you must plan how to change your lifestyle to accommodate your body's weaknesses and/or needs from a skeletal system standpoint.

Standing

The key to Posture Control Orthotic Therapy is to aid the body to become as vertical as possible. The more vertical you become, i.e., the more erect you stand, the better your posture is, the better you will feel. The less bent forward or sideways you are, the less stooped over you are, the better your physical appearance will be, but more importantly, the better you will feel physically.

Good standing posture is as follows:

1. There should be equal weight on both feet.
2. Your feet should be pointing straight or slightly outward.
3. Your knees should be straight but slightly bent, and there should be a few inches of space between them.

4. Your stomach should be pulled in.

5. Your hip and pelvic area should be tilted forward a little. Tightening your buttocks muscles helps achieve the proper pelvic position, and also flattens the lower back.

6. Stick your chest forward and out; keep your shoulders straight.

7. Hold your head high, tucking your chin in a little, and keep thinking tall, tall, tall.

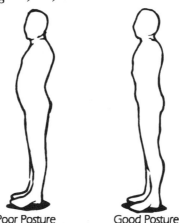

Poor Posture   Good Posture

There are really two basic keys to good standing posture. One is to keep your head held high, with your chin tucked in slightly, and the other is to make sure that your pelvis or hip area is tilted forward. This tends to flatten the lumbar spine or low back, and you will be able to maintain a good, healthy standing posture. You can use a mirror to evaluate yourself.

You should be able to maintain this erect posture whenever you are walking. Try to remember to keep your head erect, look forward and try to move smoothly, taking steps equal in length.

If you need to use walking aids such as crutches, a cane, or a walker, make sure that they are fitted properly, and that you have had proper education on how to use them. Then follow the above directions about walking as best as you can.

Standing for long periods of time in one place tends to exacerbate postural pains. If you must do so, try to change positions, i.e., bend one knee and relax on one foot for a few minutes, and then switch to the other leg. Also, if you can get a low stool, prop one foot up and then the other. Finally, make sure that your knees are not locked when you stand for any period of time.

Sitting

Sitting puts more strain on your back than standing. If you have to sit for long periods of time, you should try getting up periodically. Walk around and stretch every half-hour or so.

The chair that you choose to sit in should help you to maintain a comfortable position while using a correct sitting posture, whether you are at work or just relaxing. You should avoid slouching or bending forward in your chair. Even though this may feel good for a few minutes, it really puts a lot of strain on your back area. You should be able to sit erect and not have to lean forward when working. If possible, try sitting in a chair fifteen to thirty minutes before buying it.

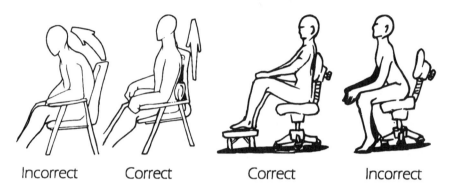

Incorrect   Correct   Correct   Incorrect

Your feet should be flat on the floor, and your low back should be well-supported. You can use a pillow, a back support, or a rolled towel to accomplish this. Your knees should be slightly higher than your hips. For this reason, an adjustable height chair is recommended. If this is not the case, you can use a book or books under your feet. This takes a lot of stress off the hips and low back area. This should also be done when positioning your seat in a car.

Your forearms should rest comfortably on the arms of your chair. Some people have congenitally short arms, and when they sit, their elbows and forearms do not reach the support of the chair. This leads to poor sitting posture and stress on your shoulders and neck. In fact, your shoulders should be relaxed if properly supported by the arm rest on the chair. If you do have short arms, then you can accommodate this condition by using foam pads or some other materials to allow the arms to rest comfortably on the chair. This is another reason why it is a good idea to have an adjustable chair.

To tell if you have short arms, stand up with your arms hanging at your sides; your elbows should reach your hips. If they are significantly higher than your hips, you probably have short arms.

If you are working at a desk, the desk height should not be too high or too low. This can cause neck and shoulder strain. You should be able to sit erect, with your shoulders relaxed slightly, and work comfortably. If you have a large desk and you have to turn a lot, you should definitely have a swivel chair, rather than twist your body frequently.

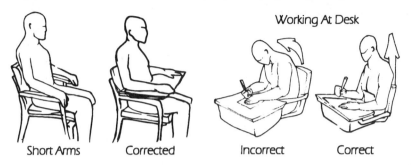

Working At Desk

Short Arms   Corrected   Incorrect   Correct

The seat cushion itself should be firm, contoured and long enough to support most of your upper legs, so as not to irritate the back of your knees. The front of the seat cushion should not sit up too high for your legs (that could also cut into and irritate the back of the knees or thigh area). Finally, if you go to athletic games such as football or basketball, which have benches without any backs, you definitely want to get a portable seat that has some cushioning and a back support to it. Sitting several hours on such a bench can put a strain on your back.

If you have had chronic back problems, it is not a good idea to sit in very low, soft cushioned couches or chairs. Besides being poor for support, it is very difficult to get out of them and this can put a lot of strain on the back.

Reading

When reading, it is very important to keep your book or paper at eye level. Many times we tend to put the materials in our lap, or we put the material on a low counter and look down while reading or writing. This puts a strain on the neck and shoulders, and certainly can perpetuate neck and shoulder postural pains. As discussed, when sitting and working at a desk, it is best to read with your head and neck fairly erect. There should be a light behind you to illuminate the material. If the light is off to the side, then you are going to have to twist your head to get better lighting, and that will put strain on your neck area.

As with sitting down, if you are going to be reading for long periods of time, then every thirty minutes or so, you should get up and change positions.

Traveling

If you are traveling by car, whether you are the driver or passenger, your body needs as much postural support as possible. This means your car seat should be in such a position that your knees are slightly bent when operating the pedals. If you are a passenger in the car, your knees should be bent also. You certainly don't want to be in a position where you have to reach to hit the pedals. This is not a good postural position, and could be dangerous as well. Many car seats do not support the lower back properly, and you may want to use a rolled up towel, a pillow or a back support. Many car seats are very soft; it is preferable to have a firm seat.

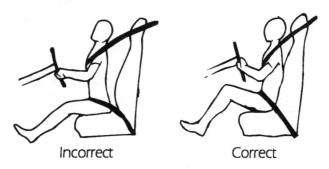

Incorrect   Correct

If you are on a long trip, you should stop frequently, at least every hour, to stretch and walk around for a few minutes. If you are traveling by plane, train or bus for a long period of time, again, while you are in the seat, you should have good body support, and this also means your knees should be a little higher than your hips. You might want to take a piece of luggage to put your feet on. You also can take some kind of support for your back. In addition, if you happen to be very tall, you may want to request an aisle seat. If you are flying on an airplane, there are certain seats, usually near the exit doors and in the first row of the cabin, that have more leg space than other seats. Again, no matter how you travel, you need to get up and walk around for a few minutes every so often.

Sleeping

Our bodies need a certain amount of rest and sleep. Obviously, if you don't sleep well, you might feel tired the next day. Also, if you sleep in an unusual position, you may end up with a "stiff neck," or back or other pain. The most important thing is to try to sleep in a position that is comfortable and is not extremely awkward. It is generally recommended that the best postural positions for sleep are either on your back, with your hips and knees bent, and a pillow under your knees, or on your side with your hips and knees bent, with a pillow between your knees. Also, if you tend to have shoulder and neck problems, you can place a pillow

between your arms while lying on
your side. You do not want to elevate
your head on too many pillows,
because that will put a strain on your
neck and shoulder muscles.
Therefore, use just one pillow if you
have a tendency towards neck and
shoulder pains. You might want to get
a specially designed pillow for these
conditions. Definitely do not sleep on
your stomach, because that puts a lot

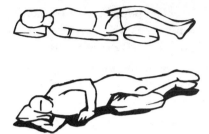

Correct Sleeping Posture

of pressure on your back. Also, if you are going to read or watch
television in your bed, try to sit fairly erect.

It is best to sleep on a good, firm mattress. Avoid a soft mattress, or
one that is old and sags, because you will not get enough support. Be
aware of how you get into and out of bed, and try to avoid any quick,
sudden movements as well as excessive twisting or bending.

If you have had chronic back problems and your bed seems to be too
soft, you can put boards of wood under your mattress for more support.
Also, some people have found it helpful to sleep on the floor at times.

Sporting Activities

There are generally three types of sporting activities: Team sports;
one-on-one competition such as tennis, boxing, and wrestling; and just
working with yourself, such as walking, running, and aerobic/dance
workouts.

This topic is covered in much more detail in Chapter 17, "The How
to of Fitness Activities." Obviously, physical conditioning, as you will note
in that chapter, is extremely important for one's overall good health.
However, if you do have postural pain/chronic pain syndromes foot to
jaw, certain activities are less likely to cause you trouble than others,
depending upon the nature of your problem and injuries. As a general
rule, the athletic activities that allow you to work within yourself or at
your own pace are usually safer. Those with the least risk often involve
walking, some swimming, slow jogging, cross country skiing, walking
machines with arm movement workouts, or similar exercises.

Sex

Restrictions on positions during sexual relations usually pertain to
people who have had recurrent chronic back problems. As with athletic
and fitness activities in general, you have to be somewhat creative in some
of the things you can and cannot do. The literature about this topic

certainly does not recommend cessation of sexual activities in most cases, with the exception being during acute bouts with back problems.

Many people, unfortunately, become frightened by the thought of having sexual relations after a prolonged or painful episode of back pain. But that need not stop them.

Essentially, the two of you should communicate, and be open-minded about what you can and cannot do. Try to make sure your back is properly supported, and avoid getting into positions that cause you pain.

Keep in mind these thoughts about the mechanics of the back area during sexual activities:

1. Try not to lie flat on your back, especially with your hips and knees rigid or straight. You can solve this problem by bending your hips and knees slightly.

2. Avoid lying on your stomach.

3. Try to control the movement or the arching of your back, which puts a lot of strain on your lower spine.

4. Do not keep your knees straight if you are going to be bending forward. By bending your knees slightly, you should be able to bend forward without any problems.

5. Not to be facetious, try to avoid any sudden twisting movements, or do the best you can.

Bending and Lifting

Bending and lifting are common, everyday actions. Because they put stress on the back, it is extremely important to be aware of certain precautions to avoid injury.

First of all, when you are going to bend down, don't bend from the waist. Bend your knees, and let them and your legs do most of the work.

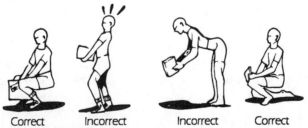

Correct   Incorrect   Incorrect   Correct

Secondly, get as close to the object as possible. Squat down as low as you can, with your feet a foot or two apart to give you stability. Then, bending your knees, try to keep your back as straight as possible. Grab whatever it is you are trying to lift, and stand up slowly. In this manner, your muscles in your legs do all the work. Then, hold the object as close to your body as you can while you are doing this. The farther away you hold it from your body, the more stress is placed on your back.

If you are moving an object from high up to put it on the ground, then follow the same techniques just mentioned, but do so in reverse order. Remember, do not try to bend down and lift something while twisting your body. Avoid any quick, sudden, jerking movements which can cause muscle strain.

While on the subject of bending, when you are sitting in a chair, do not bend over or stoop forward when getting up; this can also cause strain on your back. In addition, whenever you have to lift or carry something for any period of time, if it is possible, carry it on your back. This is much less stressful.

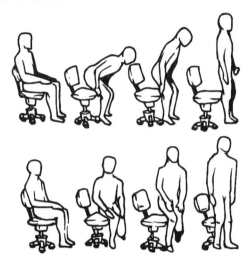

Finally, if something is extremely heavy, try to get someone to help you. Pay to hire someone now, or pay for the medical bills later.

Things to Avoid

1. Cold weather often seems to perpetuate postural pains/chronic pain syndromes. Therefore, you must dress accordingly.

2. Do not walk barefoot. As we mentioned before, one of the main functions of the feet is to absorb shock. Most people who are suffering from postural pains foot to jaw have inefficient foot and leg structure, which leads to poor shock absorption. Even if you have a six-inch- thick, cushioned carpet, there is still a hard surface underneath. So keep your shoes with your PCOs on, all the time.

3. High-heeled shoes, as we have mentioned before, may make women look better and sexier, but they certainly put a disproportionate amount of weight on the front of their feet. They put a lot of strain on the low back, and tend to make the muscles in the back of the body contract (shorten), especially the calves. From a biomechanical and skeletal system standpoint, they are a nightmare. Certainly, people who suffer from postural pains should try to wear as low-heeled shoes as possible. If you have to wear high-heeled shoes, try to rotate between one-and-a-half-inch heels one day, one-inch heels the next, and one-quarter-inch the next. In general, stay away from anything over one and one-half inches.

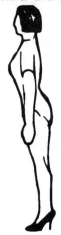

High Heels and Postural Changes

4. Try to avoid bending forward without supporting yourself properly. Bending forward or stooping to get out of a chair can strain the back, neck and shoulder areas. When getting out of a chair, try to sit erect and let your legs do the work.

5. If you tend to be on the telephone a lot, you might consider getting a headset. Certainly, at the least, you might want periodically to rotate the telephone from one side of your body to the other.

6. Clothing that is too tight can trigger certain postural pains. These include pants, belts, girdles and panty hose, which can cause circulation problems. Heavy-breasted women sometimes wear bras with straps that are too thin, and that can cause problems.

7. If you utilize a shoulder strap to carry your purse, use a briefcase regularly, or carry a child quite a lot, it would be best to rotate sides periodically.

8. There are daily activities that can cause irritations to certain muscle groups. In general, whatever it is you are doing, avoid standing too long in one place. Do not sit for hours at a time without a break. You need to get up and stretch periodically. If you are standing, sit down and relax, or lie down and stretch some. If you have a tendency to get tired because of your postural pains during daily tasks, lie down periodically and take a rest.

Incorrect   Correct

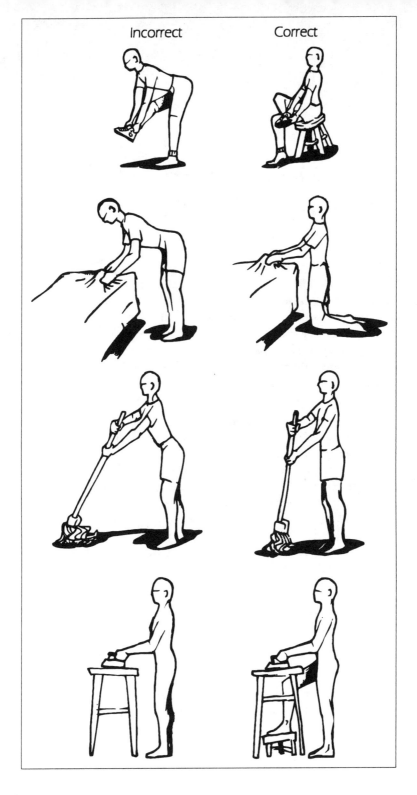

16

The How-To
Of Fitness Activities

I t is a recognized fact that good cardiovascular (heart) and pulmonary (lungs) conditioning is essential for good general health. In addition to this, people who have recurrent postural pains and chronic pain syndromes often have a problem with prolonged immobility and lack of movement of the various parts of their bodies. Prolonged immobility of these parts is often recognized as a cause of musculoskeletal system pains. Therefore, some form of repetitive, consistent movement, i.e., fitness program, is usually recommended and beneficial.

Before starting on a regular fitness program, we recommend consulting your internist, family physician, or cardiologist. In addition, if you suffer from recurrent postural pains and/or chronic pain syndromes, you may want to consult the health professional(s) who is/are treating you. There are certain basic rules for fitness and exercise training that should be followed to reduce your chances of injury and to increase your chance of success. In addition, people with chronic pain syndromes — such as myofascial pains, fibromyalgia, or recurrent postural pains — must be especially careful in pursuing fitness activities for the following reasons:

1. Not to exacerbate or actually cause a recurrence of their postural pains.

2. Not to cause a new musculoskeletal problem.

3. If done incorrectly, too quickly or too long, one might sustain an injury and give up the activity or activities.

4. A long term fitness/exercise program is a very healthy and important way to help control one's body weight. This is

very important, since overweight can contribute to perpetuating recurrent postural pain/chronic pain syndromes.

Whatever fitness activity you choose, there are certain basic principles that need to be followed:

1. You must commit yourself to a regular schedule, and give yourself enough time to get used to the activity. Starting on a program if you haven't done any exercise for a while, or if you haven't been able to due to an injury, can cause soreness in certain muscle groups in parts of your body. This is considered normal. Therefore, we recommend that you give yourself six months before you make any judgments about giving up or changing the activity.

2. You should outline a very achievable, well-thought-out program with realistic goals. Set your program up so that you can reach certain goals within a sensible time. This will build up your self-confidence, help motivate you to continue, and diminish your chance of injury or disappointment. For example, if you are going to start a walking program, then you may just go and walk five or ten minutes at a very leisurely pace every other day for two weeks. Then you should increase your distance gradually, i.e., two to five minutes or one-half mile every other day, every two weeks, until you are continuously walking for thirty minutes or so, three to four days a week. Once you reach the thirty minute plateau, you can pick up the pace if you want to, but again, gradually.

3. Never increase the distance and pace at the same time. Do one or the other. It is usually recommended to lengthen distance first, and then the pace. For walking, after you have gotten up to at least thirty minutes, you could cut your pace per mile by five to fifteen seconds every two to four weeks. Do not attempt to do this for every single mile walked in a particular week. The sensible percentage would be about 20 to 25 percent of your total weekly mileage.

   If you are lifting weights, increase the number of repetitions first. After a few weeks, gradually increase the weight itself. Do not do both at once.

4. A key point to remember is that it is necessary to stress your body slightly beyond its current capability, so that it will grow stronger. To be successful in such a program, a fitness person must be able to handle stress consistently.

5. It is very important not to push yourself too far, too fast, too soon. This will only drain you physically, lead to injury, be emotionally depressing, and could defeat your purpose.

To reach good cardiovascular fitness levels, you must exercise for at least thirty minutes three to four times a week. Three days is definitely the minimum. It is ideal to elevate your heart rate to 70 to 85 percent of its maximum for this period of time. If you are overweight, diabetic, have led a sedentary existence, or have had a debilitating disease, 60 to 70 percent would be more appropriate, certainly for the first six months.

Figure Your Heart Rate:

- To obtain your maximum heart rate, subtract your age from 220.

- Then take your pulse by placing your second and third fingers gently on the underside of either wrist. Count the number of beats in fifteen seconds and multiply this figure by four. This will give your the number of beats per minute. Taking your pulse via the carotid artery in the neck (on either side of the Adam's Apple), is not recommended because it is not as accurate. Check your pulse regularly during your program (every fifteen minutes or so) to be sure you are attaining the proper target heart rate range. As your fitness level improves and you get more accustomed to your body's signals, you won't have to check as often, unless you want to.

- Caution: you should not exceed 85 percent of your maximum heart rate for any workout.

For example, if you are 50 years of age, you would calculate the maximum heart rate as follows: 220 minus 50 equals 170; 70 percent of 170 is approximately 119. Therefore, a pulse rate of 119 or higher per thirty minutes would indicate a hard workout. Caution: you should never exceed 85 percent of your maximum heart rate for any workout. In this case, 85 percent equals 144.

6. Five minutes after finishing exercising, your pulse should be below 120/110 if 50 or over. Your heart rate should be under 100 beats per minute after ten minutes or so, and back to a normal resting pulse in thirty minutes. Check this. If this is not the case, you are overtrained, or something may be wrong. If concerned or in doubt, you may want to seek professional advice.

7. You should not train hard more than three days of the week, and an easy or rest day must follow every hard workout, no matter how many different types of fitness activities are involved. They may each use different muscles, but you have just one heart.

8. You must be flexible; always remember to listen to your body. Do not become rigid with your program. If you feel tired, didn't get enough sleep, realize the weather might be hazardous, or you just don't feel like it one day, DON'T. Or go out slowly, take it easy, cut back on your distance or pace. When in doubt, take it slow, cut back.

9. You may need to get more sleep or adjust your diet, because as you improve or get more involved with fitness activities, your energy needs may increase. If your responsibilities at work pile up, or if you are under excessive emotional stress, you may have to cut back in your fitness program. This could and should be only temporary, but it needs to be addressed, or it could lead to injury.

10. Since the idea for most of us is to have fun and try to increase our fitness at the same time, you should feel refreshed after most of your daily workouts, after a period of adjustment of several months.

11. You should warm up properly before your activity. This means you should stretch 10 minutes prior to your starting. Start out at a slower pace for the first minute or two. This allows the muscles in your body to warm up properly and be ready for your workout. After your fitness activity, it is best to slow down for the last five minutes, to cool the body down. Here again, you should try to stretch afterwards. However, if you are too rushed to stretch, then do a second stretch routine later on in the evening. You are better off not doing it at all if you are doing it incorrectly or rushed. There are several good books available on stretching as it relates to different fitness activities/sports. Consult one of these to get information about which ones and how to do them properly for whatever activity or activities you are participating in.

12. It is a good idea to keep a record or "log" of your fitness program. Record such things as:

    • how many weeks or months you have been at it.

    • how long or far.

    • how fast and/or intensity.

- what fitness shoes you used, if appropriate, and/or equipment.
- how you felt before and after.
- how high your pulse rate went.

This information can be useful to you in several ways. It will serve as a monitor of your progress, and, in case of injury or setback, could be an invaluable tool to help you understand your injury. It may even prevent a new or recurring one! It can also be used as a motivational tool, to see how far you've come.

13. Overtraining. Overdoing it is a major cause of fitness injuries. Your body will usually send you signals or warnings that you are overdoing it. Following are some hints about how you can determine if you are overtraining.

   a. Take your pulse every morning before getting out of bed. Rest in bed for a minute or so after waking up, and take your resting pulse. Do this every day and record it in your training log. After two weeks or so, you will get an average resting pulse. If your pulse is 7 to 10 beats higher on a particular morning, then you should consider a day off, or at least cut back on the duration and/or the intensity of your workout. Perhaps a few days off is indicated. Cut back until your pulse returns to normal.

   There may be some emotional reasons your pulse is faster than normal. There may be something exciting or stressful in your personal life. This naturally increases the pulse rate. If this is the case, you might disregard the need to take it easy. Perhaps a workout, such as walking, running, or bicycle riding, will do you good and reduce the stress.

   b. Your pulse should return to normal no longer than 30 minutes after a workout. If it has not, this indicates (at least) an overtrained body.

   c. Record your daily weight, especially if you are into heavy distance training. This is more important in warm weather, outdoor activities. A weight loss of three or more pounds overnight usually means an injury or illness in two or three days.

   d. Urine is supposed to be clear and odorless. In a dehydrated, overstressed athlete, it will be darker and perhaps have an odor; blood may even appear.

e. Unusually thirsty after a workout? Are you drinking more fluids than usual? If so, this can indicate a potential problem two or three days later.

f. Sleeping habits should be considered. Going to bed later than normal increases the chance of injury. A decreased number in the hours of sleep, plus broken, frequently interrupted sleep, is also a negative sign.

The Overuse Syndrome

The overuse syndrome is usually an indication of overtraining.

- tired or fatigued during normal daily activities.

- bushed or drained of energy when trying to get through a day after a fitness workout.

- nagging tightness, aches and pains, especially in the muscles.

- difficulty falling asleep, or waking often in the middle of the night and inability to fall back asleep; difficulty waking up in the morning.

- headaches, frequent colds, or flu-like symptoms, despite no actual fever or illness.

- losing the desire to train (do you feel like you are going stale all of a sudden?).

- recurrent fever blisters on your lips; irregular menstrual cycle in women.

- changes in bowel movement habits (diarrhea or constipation).

Listen to your body. Many of us have sustained sport injuries. These old injured areas often ache and become tight when we overstress our bodies. If you have had a past injury, then at least use it in a positive way. If it acts up, take it easy.

These are all signs and symptoms of the overuse syndrome, indicating overtraining. If you have some of these signs, then you are probably overtrained, and should take it easy or rest for a few days, or at least until the feelings and symptoms subside. Re-evaluate your training schedule, so as not to overdo it again. Make sure you have enough time, or are allowing enough time to warm up, stretch properly, and cool down properly. When you resume your fitness activity, do so at a lesser level than you were and gradually build up again.

Remember: No schedule is perfect. There are many variables to deal with and despite careful adherence to a seemingly gradual, sound program, an injury may still occur.

14. Whatever activity you want to participate in, you must make sure your posture is correct while doing it, whether walking, cycling, lifting weights, or any other exercise. If in doubt, seek the advice of your health care professional, a personal trainer, an experienced fitness person and/or books, magazines, and videos.

15. You must have appropriate equipment. If you want to do walking as an exercise, use walking shoes. If outdoors, dress accordingly. If you want to do aerobics, use aerobic shoes. If you cycle, make sure the seat is adjusted properly, and so on.

> Don't forget that it is better to take your time increasing your fitness levels. If you go too far, too fast, too soon and too frequently, you will most likely be sorry. When in doubt, moderation is the word.

Special Advice for Chronic Pain Syndrome People

In addition to following the basic training principles of fitness already described, people who suffer recurrent postural pains/chronic pain syndromes should also heed the following advice.

1. You must consult with your health care professional or someone he/she recommends to you, when getting involved with a fitness program. Physical therapists and/or personal trainers, who have experience with these types of problems, can be very helpful.

2. At least initially, it is very important to work one-on-one with one of these professionals. Modification on how you go about a specific fitness activity is often needed because of certain physical limitations that recurrent postural pains/chronic pain syndrome people have.

3. Proper form, as previously mentioned, is important to reduce the chance of injury for all of us, but it cannot be emphasized enough here. These types of people often have restricted ranges of motion of certain joints and very tight or weakened muscles that require modified movements and techniques to overcome them.

   Most people in fitness activities either start on their own, or, even when doing it through various health clubs and other fitness centers, tend to lift weights and use postural positions that are not correct. If they are fortunate enough not to be a chronic pain person, they can often get away with this. But if you are a chronic pain person, you must be extra careful.

4. Some of the more aggressive fitness activities, such as running, high impact aerobics, basketball, football, and wrestling are too rough, have too much shock impacted to the body, and are contraindicated. The best overall activity to gain endurance would be a walking program. It has minimal needs and equipment. It is much less stressful, in terms of shock generated to the body, compared to most other activities. Walking can be done either inside on a treadmill, in a shopping mall, indoor track, or outside in mild weather. Cold weather can trigger a lot of recurrent postural pains/chronic pain syndromes. If you prefer to exercise outdoors, you must dress warmly to protect your body and the particular joints/muscles that are susceptible to chronic problems.

    Depending on the severity of your condition(s), very low-impact aerobics, cycling and walking machines are good exercise alternatives.

5. Cross training is often recommended. This prevents spending too much time in one position, which can often lead to stiffness and pain. For example, if you have worked up to forty minutes of continuous exercise, and all of it was cycling on a stationary bike (which is usually less stressful on the back), you may get stiff from being in this one position too long. This may cause you pain and limit your fitness program in and of itself. You would be better off cycling for ten to fifteen minutes, getting up and stretching a little, then walking for ten to fifteen minutes, stretching again, and finishing up cycling, or spending a few minutes on a walking machine or lifting weights.

Weak Muscles

Many people with recurrent postural pains/chronic pain syndromes often have weak muscle groups around joints and parts of their bodies that give them ongoing problems. If that is the case, your health professional may recommend that weight exercises be utilized in order to strengthen these muscles. These muscles should be exercised using light weights, with repetitions. This must be done very carefully, with instruction on form by a knowledgeable professional. Increasing the repetitions should be done very slowly, so as not to exacerbate the original problem(s). It is also important to be able to take the muscle groups involved through a complete range of motion. Partial ranges of motion tend to contribute to chronic pain syndromes and perpetuate them. Jerky and rapid start-and-stop movements can also overstress muscles.

Stretching

Chronic pain people often are very stiff when they get out of bed in the morning and after sitting for long periods of time. If this is the case, specific stretching or flexibility exercises are often recommended for the muscle group(s) involved. Ideally, these should be done before you get out of bed and after you sit for long periods of time, to loosen the muscles before getting up. It is extremely important to stretch the muscles several times a day. It is also a good idea to do stretching after your body is warm. This means doing at least one good stretching program daily, after a bath, shower, using a Jacuzzi or the use of a heating pad to warm the area(s) up, or some liniment ointment that produces heat.

1. Try to be completely relaxed when stretching.
2. Rhythmic breathing is extremely effective in inducing relaxation.
3. There should be no jerky motion or movement in your stretch.
4. The stretch should be done slowly.
5. There should be no burning or pain caused by the stretch. If you begin to feel these, this is as far as you should go. Then, hold that for ten to twenty seconds, then try to go a little further, as you feel the muscles giving. Then you hold it for another twenty seconds, then stretch a little further, if you can, and hold it for an additional twenty seconds. I recommend each stretch be done twice, with a few seconds rest in between.
6. If a stretch causes pain that lasts after the exercise, it should be avoided for awhile.
7. Stretching should be done on an individual basis. Some of us are more flexible then others. Certainly, if you have suffered recurrent postural pains/chronic pain syndromes, this is the case. Do not force yourself to do what someone else can, because your body may not allow it.

Special Postural Collapse Stretching

As mentioned previously, postural collapse leads to tight muscles in the front of the body, and overstretched, weakened muscles in the back. Stretches that promote flexibility in the muscle groups listed below are often recommended. It is important to note that a qualified health care professional, with expertise in exercise and the chronic pain patient, should usually be involved. The reason for this is that, if done incorrectly, stretching will not only be ineffective, but can make matters worse.

The muscle groups are:

1. The front and sides of the neck.
2. The front and sides of the chest.
3. The stomach muscles.
4. The outside of the upper and lower legs.
5. The front of the lower legs.

It is important to note that each person (patient) may have different variations that must and should be addressed individually.

There are numerous written and visual resources available that demonstrate how to stretch specific muscle groups.

17

When You're Pregnant

I t seems like most, if not all, women who are pregnant experience back pain at some point in time. Most seem to expect this as part of the program, so to speak. There are really three reasons why, during pregnancy, this seems to occur.

First of all, most women start to feel very tired and need more rest from the first trimester on. Therefore, they may start to become less active than they once were. This comparatively sedentary existence leads to a general muscle weakness because of disuse. That is, the muscles tend to get out of shape. Then, after a few months, a weight gain occurs, mostly in the stomach area. The burden of this change in your body really lays on the spine, low back, and to some extent, your feet and legs. The muscles, tendons, ligaments and joints of the feet up through the back are placed under excessive strains. They fatigue more easily, can go into spasms and eventually can cause pain. Finally, during the third trimester, a hormone is released (called relaxin) that leads to ligament laxity. That means a weakness develops in the ligaments in your body. This hormone is released in order to allow for pelvic expansion that is needed for birth. But it can affect ligaments everywhere else in the body.

Added to all this is the fact that most people are born with varying degrees of excessive pronation. If no other variables were present, which is *not* the case, then some women with mild excessive pronation would theoretically have none to mild low back problems. Someone with moderate excessive pronation would suffer more, and someone with severe excessive pronation would have a greater tendency towards back problems, and the severity of the pain would be even greater.

Many other variables come into play, such as the actual amount of weight gained, the type of work or chores done daily, the amount of time a woman has to be on her feet, the amount of lifting done daily (lifting other children, occupational requirements), types of shoes one wears, the type of surface one walks on, and other such factors.

Another way of looking at it is that between the muscle disuse, the weight gain and inherent weakness of the body's ligaments, someone who is only a mild pronator, for this period of time, becomes a moderate pronator. A moderate pronator becomes a severe pronator. A severe pronator becomes a more severe pronator. Since excessive pronation, in and of itself, can lead to postural pains, it is no wonder that back problems are so prevalent during pregnancy.

You do not necessarily have to assume that you are going to suffer from back problems during pregnancy. There are several things you can do to try to avoid it. First of all, it is important that you consult with your OB/GYN before considering any exercise program. Normally, if there are no complications precluding it, then a regular exercise program would be indicated, with special emphasis on trying to strengthen the low back and abdominal muscles as much as possible. Secondly, you should try to be aware of maintaining a good erect posture. Also, minimize the stress you place on your back and legs. This has to do with the way you stand, sit, and bend. See Chapter 15, "Position Is Everything — Sitting, Standing, Sleeping, Sex, Etc.," for more information.

In addition, try to find time to rest, preferably lying down periodically during the day, to get the strain off your skeletal system, especially your back. You should not go barefoot when walking on a hard surface, and you should wear good supportive, shock-absorbing shoes. Try to stay away from high-heeled shoes completely, if possible.

Posture Control Orthotics have proven to be very successful in compensating for excessive pronation, which is certainly exacerbated during pregnancy. Therefore, the end result of low back pain and/or leg and foot problems associated with pregnancy can often be dramatically reduced and even eliminated.

Obviously, there is a percentage of pregnant women who suffer from recurrent postural pain/chronic pain syndromes. If you are one, you must be extremely careful in trying to adhere to the necessary adjustments and requirements for daily living, in order to reduce the chances of perpetuating/exacerbating your problems. You must also be aware that you are more apt to have problems during pregnancy than someone who does not have these problems to begin with.

18

Your Psychological Outlook

One's psychological outlook can have a profound effect on perpetuating and/or overcoming postural pain/chronic pain syndromes foot to jaw. There are at least six different aspects of how one's emotional well being can affect these painful conditions.

1. Excessive stress, tension and anxiety can be a major contributing factor to musculoskeletal disorders because muscles get very tense and tight when we are stressed.

2. Your psychological outlook can play a significant role in your ability to recover or overcome postural pains foot to jaw. Inability to cope with excessive stress, tension, anxiety and depression could definitely impede your ability to heal, and certainly slow down your rate of recovery.

3. People who have recurrent chronic pain syndromes foot to jaw for years and years are often very anxious and under a lot of stress because they constantly have to deal with the pain physically and emotionally, day in and day out. In a sense, many of them are afraid of living, afraid to perform everyday activities, which they fear may perpetuate or cause pain and lead to hospitalization or surgery. So they have a lot of psychological reasons to be uptight and upset. This is a vicious cycle, because the tension only perpetuates the chronic pain.

4. On the other hand, there are people who develop a macho attitude about their problem(s). They will force themselves and their bodies, and not attempt to adjust or cut back in any way. They forge ahead, and are constantly stressing their already tired, weak and/or injured body.

Consequently, they are inhibiting, or slowing down, their ability to heal.

5. There are those people who actually have psychosomatic postural pains/chronic pain syndromes foot to jaw. Estimates are that as high as 40 percent of low back pain suffers could be considered in this category. The reasons for this can vary, but often are related to someone's not wanting to make or face a very important decision. Another situation is where someone has to do something that is very frightening to them, especially for the first time. An example of this is someone who is contemplating having to go far away from home for a long period of time.

6. Some people find that having these recurrent/chronic painful conditions gets them a good deal of attention that they never had before, and they do not want that to end.

7. Finally, there are those who have financial reasons for not getting well. These are people involved in workmen's compensation injury cases and lawsuits.

For those people in categories 1, 2, 3 and 4 above, trying to learn relaxation techniques in order to help cope with tension and anxiety in their daily lives would certainly prove invaluable. There are many books written on this topic, as well as chronic pain support groups of various types available to them. When indicated, professional counseling could be helpful.

For people in categories 5 and 6, it is important to remember that no matter what the cause of the so-called psychosomatic illnesses, they do experience real pain, whether related to trauma or not. Therefore, they should not be disregarded or looked down upon, but are often in need of professional counseling and help.

It is a well-documented fact that many postural pain/chronic pain syndromes can be exacerbated and perpetuated by anxiety and mental stress. Stressful situations, whether good or bad, cause certain physical changes within our bodies. We tend to tense up, and our muscles can become tight. Our bodies can usually handle this without any negative effects for a short period. However, if we never get a chance to relax or release the tension, if there is no outlet for the stress, it can end up hurting us physically.

19

Physical Therapy Treatments To Do At Home

M any people who suffer from recurrent postural pain/chronic pain syndromes foot to jaw often are expected to do various forms of home exercise, massage and treatment for themselves.

> Self-treatment, as discussed in this book, is not recommended for people who have diabetes, circulatory problems, acute infections, poor eyesight, or allergies to ice or heat. If you fit into this category, then seek professional advice before proceeding.

Depending upon your problem and situation, you may at one time or another want to utilize cold, hot and massage therapies.

Ice Treatments

The use of cold causes vascular constriction, that is, it decreases the size (width) of blood vessels to an area, and thus helps in controlling immediate swelling and reducing pain. Cold therapy should be used immediately after an injury to an area. It should be applied approximately 20 minutes, and then left off the area for 20 minutes, for at least a few hours. If you are bedridden because you are injured, you can use the ice treatments over the first 24 to 48 hours.

Initially, when ice is applied to the area, it feels very cold; after a few minutes, it starts to hurt and feel achy. The area eventually gets numb.

> Caution: Some people are allergic to cold, break out in hives and actually have pain. If you are one of these people, consult with a health care professional before using .

Another use for cold therapy is if you have an injury or a postural problem, but it is not severe enough to stop you from doing your daily activities. Cold can be used to reduce the swelling and/or discomfort. You should elevate and ice the area(s) involved, 20 minutes on and 20 minutes off.

There are different types of cold modalities available at home. Which one you use will be dependent on what is available to you at the time, and which area(s) of the body you wish to ice down:

1. Ice cubes placed in an ice bag or a makeshift ice bag (a plastic bag covered by a towel, so the ice is not applied directly on the skin)

2. Reusable cold packs can be bought in a store and can be refrozen.

3. Buckets of cold water with 5 to 10 ice cubes, for icing down the hands and feet, or a bathtub filled with ice cubes, so the temperature is about 55 to 65 degrees Fahrenheit and can be used for larger areas of the body.

4. A paper cup filled with water, then placed in the freezer so that it becomes a frozen cube, can be utilized for ice massage therapy. You take the frozen cup out of the freezer, peel away the top layer of the cup, and use it to massage an area.

Heat Treatments

Heat causes vascular dilation, that is, it increases the width of blood vessels in an area. This is usually applied after initial inflammation has receded. Heat increases blood supply to an area, and, therefore, aids in the removal of damaged tissue from the area, promoting healing. Heat should be utilized twenty to thirty minutes, three or four times daily. If you have recently overcome a rather severe injury, then the body part being treated with heat may have to be elevated during this time.

Another way heat is utilized is to warm up an area or areas of your body before doing a fitness activity, daily chores or occupational requirements. In this application, heat should be applied for about five to ten minutes.

Recurrent postural pain/chronic pain syndrome patients are often required, or expected, to do home stretching exercises after heating the involved area(s). This is best done after taking a shower or a bath. If this is not possible, use a heating pad or a heat producing ointment as a last choice.

The type of heat source you use depends upon what is available and what part or parts of the body you want to use it on.

1. Heating pad should have an external cover over it. If not, put a towel over it, so it is not directly against the skin. It should be used on the medium setting.

2. For applications of deep heat, do the following: Caution: YOU SHOULD ONLY USE HEATING PADS DESIGNATED FOR HOME USE WITH MOIST HEAT. Apply a steaming hot towel, for approximately one or two minutes over the area involved. Repeat this two times, then apply a heat producing ointment or liniment to the area; then reapply two applications of the steaming hot towel as mentioned above. After a few minutes, the towel will have cooled down. Then apply a heating pad over the area on medium setting for 15 to 20 minutes. This type of heat application should be done three or four times daily, if possible.

3. Warm water baths are also very relaxing and useful when trying to help treat recurrent chronic postural pains foot to jaw. The bath temperature should be around 90 to 105 degrees Fahrenheit.

4. Home Jacuzzis, or whirlpools, are extremely useful because they combine heat with massage. This is excellent for people who have chronic pain conditions. This should be done for about 20 minutes daily.

Massage

Massage is hands-on rubbing or kneading of body tissues to relax muscles, promote healing, and increase circulation. This helps reduce fluids which accumulate in an injured area. Massage techniques also reduce scar tissue and/or adhesions. Depending upon the area(s), common massage techniques can be done to yourself, or you can have someone do the massage on you. There are books, videos and other sources of information available that teach the different types of massage techniques.

Also, electrical vibrators/massage units of varying sizes and shapes can be bought. They can also be very useful to knead or massage tight, achy muscles.

Home Exercise Programs

Home exercise programs are often recommended and expected of people with recurrent postural pains/chronic pain syndromes foot to jaw. These exercises are recommended to be done after heat is applied to the area. See Chapter 16, "The How-To of Fitness Activities," for more information.

R.I.C.E.

As you know, this book is mainly written for people who have recurrent postural pains foot to jaw. However, there are certain times when acute flare-ups of pain or injury/injuries may occur. If this is the case, then the initial treatment recommended is called RICE.

R = Rest

I = Ice

C = Compression (the area being treated should be compressed, using some type of bandaging if possible)

E = Elevation (the area being treated, should be elevated above the level of the heart)

The different elements that are included in RICE are aimed at reducing initial swelling and pain. Once swelling and pain is under control, which usually takes about 24 to 48 hours, heat treatments can be started, as described previously.

Orthopedic Supports

There are many products available to help you support or brace different parts of your body. You might want to consult with your health care professional if you have a recurrent postural pain/chronic pain syndrome foot to jaw, because it is advisable to exercise some areas and to brace others.

The supports range from ankle supports, knee supports, knee braces and back supports or braces, to elbow, wrist and hand supports. There are special types of shoulder harnesses or supports available, and specially designed cervical pillows and cervical wraps to help support the neck and head area. There is also a combination cervical and shoulder wrap support.

There are stores and catalogues that offer types of furniture which can be useful to you, such as chairs for both working and relaxing, and portable desk slants that can be attached to chairs and desks. Special footrests, ottomans, arm supports for chairs, low back support cushions or car seats, upholstered sofas, rockers, and massage chairs are also available. In addition, there are special types of beds and mattresses. There are mats for people who have to stand in one place for long periods of time, such as cashiers and hair dressers. For more information about these kinds of supports, or furniture, look in the phone book under orthopedic supplies, or call your health care professional.

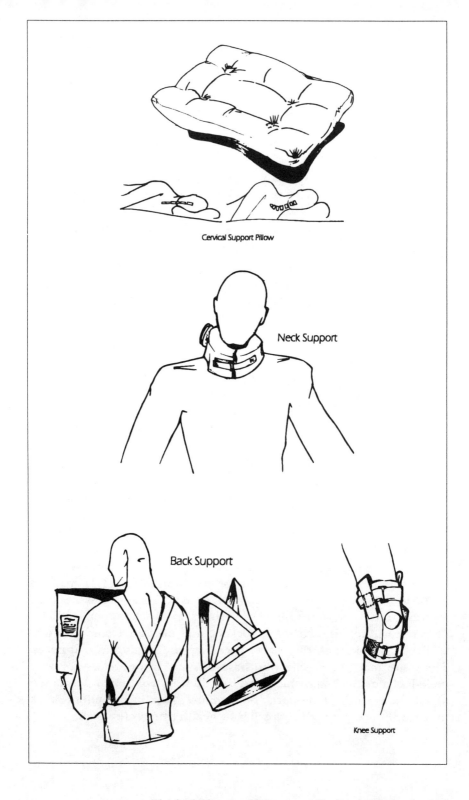

Cervical Support Pillow

Neck Support

Back Support

Knee Support

Appendix I

Results of Subjective Outcome Studies

Three separate subjective outcome studies were analyzed, one year after completion of therapy. The chief complaint had been either knee, back, or neck pain. The results of these studies follow. They demonstrate that excessive foot pronation, secondary to forefoot varum, can contribute to chronic postural pains foot to jaw. More importantly, they also show how Posture Control Orthotic Therapy often can control body mechanics and improve chronic knee, back and neck pains respectively.

These studies were conducted by Brian A. Rothbart, DPM, Ph.D., and Kathleen Yerratt, R.N., at the Bellevue Foot and Ankle Center in Bellevue, Washington.

Knee Study

One hundred twenty-eight chronic knee pain patients who had been treated with PCOs participated in a three-year subjective follow-up study from 1989 to 1992.

All these patients had been treated, prior to PCOs, with various modalities (anti-inflammatory medications, aggressive physical therapy, surgery). Results had been disappointing. Attenuation of pain and disability had not met patient expectations. All of these patients were professionally advised that "nothing else could be done." Many were referred to pain management facilities to learn how to cope with their pain and live with their disability. This coping process is termed *body hardening.*

One year after PCO therapy was concluded, questionnaires were sent to each of one hundred twenty-eight patients. The participants were asked to evaluate the percentage of knee improvement since wearing PCOs. Of one hundred twenty-eight respondents, eight reported an improved range of improvement of ten to forty percent. Fourteen improved fifty to sixty percent, and *seventy-eight reported improvement of seventy percent or greater.* Twenty-five respondents reported improvement, with no range given. One reported no improvement, and two reported their knee symptoms increased.

Conclusion: Excessive pronation secondary to forefoot varum deformity can contribute to chronic knee pain. Postural Control Orthotic Therapy can successfully control body mechanics and improve knee symptoms in most cases.

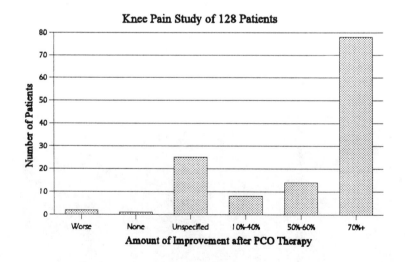

Knee Pain Study of 128 Patients

Low Back Pain Study

Excessive foot pronation, with triplane talar deviation and calcaneal eversion, is frequently observed in chronic pain patients. Clinical data strongly suggests that decreasing this excessive pronation can dramatically reduce joint symptoms.

In a recent clinical study, two hundred eight patients with chronic low back pain were treated with Postural Control Orthotic Therapy. All of these patients had had unrelenting pain, which was rarely related to trauma. All of the patients had been previously treated unsuccessfully by multiple practitioners.

The following subjective outcomes were reported one year after completion of therapy: Nineteen of the two hundred eight patients reported total resolution of their low back pain with Postural Control Orthotic Therapy. *One hundred twenty of the two hundred eight patients reported between seventy and ninety percent subjective improvement in their low back symptoms.* Thirty-seven of the patients reported between forty and sixty percent subjective improvement; eighteen patients reported between ten and thirty percent improvement; and six patients reported no improvement in their subjective symptoms. Three patients reported an exacerbation of their back pain. Overall, more than ninety percent of the patients participating in this study improved.

Forefoot Varum deformity was identified in two hundred two of the two hundred eight patients treated. The six patients without a forefoot varum deformity reported either a worsening or no improvement in their low back symptoms.

Conclusion: Excessive pronation secondary to forefoot varum deformity can contribute to chronic low back pain. Postural Control Orthotic Therapy can successfully control body mechanics and improve low back symptoms in most cases.

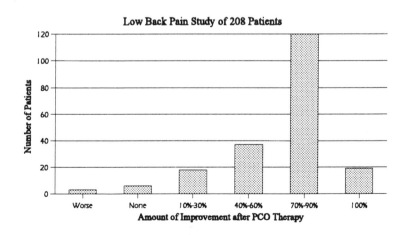

Low Back Pain Study of 208 Patients

Neck Pain Study

Excessive foot pronation, with triplane talar deviation and calcaneal eversion, is frequently observed in chronic pain patients. Clinical data strongly suggests that decreasing this excessive pronation will dramatically reduce joint symptoms.

In a recent clinical study, seventy-three patients with chronic neck pain were treated with Postural Control Orthotics. All of these patients had had unrelenting pain which was rarely related to a specific injury. All of the patients had been previously treated unsuccessfully by multiple practitioners.

The following subjective outcomes were reported one year after completion of therapy: Four of the seventy-three patients reported total resolution of their neck pain with Postural Control Orthotic (PCO) therapy. *Thirty-two of the seventy-three patients reported between seventy and ninety percent subjective improvement in their neck symptoms.* Nineteen patients reported between forty and sixty percent subjective improvement; eight patients reported between ten and thirty percent improvement; and two patients reported no improvement in their subjective symptoms. None of the patients reported an exacerbation of their neck pain. Overall, more than ninety percent of the patients participating in this study improved.

Forefoot Varum deformity was identified in seventy-one of the seventy-three patients treated. The two patients without a forefoot varum deformity proved intractable to Posture Control Orthotic Therapy.

Excessive foot and ankle pronation, secondary to forefoot varum deformity, can contribute to chronic neck pain. Postural Control Orthotic Therapy can successfully control body mechanics and improve chronic neck symptoms in most cases.

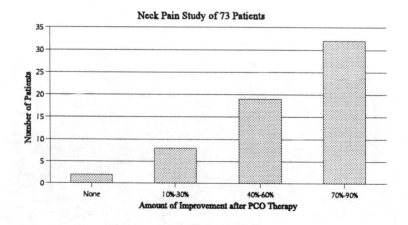

Neck Pain Study of 73 Patients

Appendix II

How To Seek Posture Control Orthotic Therapy

PCO, Inc., is a professional orthotic company dedicated to the clinical application of mechanical medicine and the resolution of postural pains and chronic pain syndromes foot to jaw. By using mechanical engineering principles, a highly sophisticated orthotic, called a Posture Control Orthotic, was developed. It proved to have a profound influence on the body's biomechanics and postural alignment.

These Posture Control Orthotics have been found to be extremely effective in reducing subjective symptoms associated with postural pains and chronic pain syndromes foot to jaw. More importantly, they have allowed for ongoing resolution of such pains.

Posture Control Orthotic Therapy has been utilized by many different types of medical professionals, including physicians in pain management facilities, physical medicine and rehabilitation physicians, osteopaths, chiropractors, dentists who specialize in cranial mandibular orthopedics, podiatrists, naturalists, physical and massage therapists, and others to date.

For more information, please write to me at 7540 Little River Turnpike, Annandale, VA (22203).

Glossary

Abducted - a part of the body is drawn away from the midline of the body.

Achilles Tendon - the large tendon just above and in back of the heel. It connects the calf (gastrocsoleus) muscles to the back of the heel bone (calcaneus).

Adducted - a part of the body is drawn towards the midline of the body.

Anemia - insufficient quality or quantity of red blood cells.

Ankylosing Spondylitis - a chronic, progressive arthritic disease of young men. Its cause is unknown; it usually affects the spinal and sacroiliac joints, leading to fusion and deformity.

Anterior Chain - muscles in the front of the body.

Arch Supports - devices worn in shoes, under the feet, primarily designed to support the arch. They are usually not custom made to an individual's foot, and are available commercially.

Arthritis - inflammation of a joint.

Biomechanics - the study of the dynamic musculoskeletal system of the human being; how it functions and moves.

Asymmetrical - not equal, not the same. Different.

Biomechanical Exam - examination of the dynamic musculoskeletal system of the body.

BioShim - a wedge of material that allows for the application of vertical height in dress shoes for men and women.

BioVector a triangular shaped device with a scale marked across the top and sides. The scale represents vertical height from the ground in millimeters. It measures forefoot and rearfoot varum.

Body Hardening - a process whereby people who suffer from recurrent postural pain/chronic pain syndromes are taught how to cope and live with their pains and disability/disabilities.

Boney Ankle Equinus - limitation of movement of the foot towards the leg at the ankle joint due to a boney enlargement or fusion.

Boney fusion - joining bones together.

Bowlegged - also known as genu varum. When standing, the legs are curving outwards, the knees are apart more than is considered normal and the ankles are touching or are very close together.

Bursa - a soft tissue sac of fluid that acts as a lubricant. Located between body parts that move upon one another. Often found between bones and muscles.

Bursitis - inflammation of a bursa.

Calibrate - to measure.

Calibration - measuring .

Cancer - any disease characterized by malignant tumor formation or proliferation (rapid and increased growth) of a more primitive form of fully developed cells.

Cardiologist - a physician who specializes in the diagnosis and treatment of disorders of the heart.

CAT Scan - a special X-ray test, Computerized Axial Tomography, which involves the simultaneous taking of many X-rays from multiple angles. Results in a highly defined set of pictures of a body organ or organs.

Cervical - pertaining to the neck.

Chiropractor - a person who practices a branch of healing that believes that most diseases are caused by nerve compression resulting from faulty vertebrae alignment.

Chronic Pain Syndrome - long-term, unrelenting pain experienced in various parts of their body from the feet to the legs, knees, hips, back, neck, shoulder, jaw and head. Typical scenario for these patients is various types of treatments, such as manual medicine, physical therapy, oral anti-inflammatory medication, muscle relaxants, painkillers, steroid injections, and trigger point injections. Many are referred for psychotherapy, given anti-depressants, nutritional counseling, or weight control. Often, one or combinations of these therapies work, but for short periods of time and/or as long as therapy continues. Afterward, there is a cycle downward.

Coccyx - the tail bone. The last bone of the spinal column.

Compensated- a change in one part of the body to adjust or makeup for an abnormal force, structure or position and/or inefficient functioning of another part of the body.

Conventional Orthotics - usually custom-made devices worn in shoes under the feet. They not only support the arch of the foot in midstance, but also can reduce early stance phase (heel contact) excessive pronation.

Cranial Mandibular Orthopedics - the diagnosis and treatment of musculoskeletal disorders that affect the head, jaw and facial areas of the body.

Deviation - departure from what is considered normal or standard.

126

Double Support - when both feet are in contact with the ground at the same time. Occurs for two brief periods of time during the total gait cycle.

Dysfunctional - abnormal or impaired functioning.

Equinus - limitation of the movement of the foot towards the leg at the ankle joint.

Eversion - turning outward of a part of the body or structure from the midline of the body.

Everted -a part of the body is turned outward from the midline of the body.

Excessive Pronation - pronation in excess of what is considered normal, which is about four to six degrees.

Fetus - the unborn child during pregnancy.

Forefoot Varum - the inside front of the foot (the ball) is angled (twisted) from the ground.

Gait - also referred to as walking. Repetitive acts of one's body falling forward, and then one's foot contacting the ground and catching one's self. In the meantime, the opposite foot and leg are moving off the ground.

Gait Analysis - the analysis/evaluation of walking.

Gait Cycle - the time it takes from when the heel of one's foot contacts the walking surface to when the heel of the same foot contacts the walking surface again.

Genu Valgum - also known as knock-kneed. When standing, the bones of the legs are bending inward, the knees are touching or very close together, and the ankles are apart more than considered normal.

Genu Varum - also known as bowlegged. When standing the legs are curving outwards, the knees are apart more than is considered normal, and the ankles are touching or are very close together.

Gout - a type of arthritis or inflammation around a joint, caused by excessive uric acid in the blood. Attacks occur suddenly and are accompanied by redness, swelling and pain.

Gravity - the pull on all bodies in the earth's sphere toward the earth's center.

Heel Contact - the first part of the stance phase of gait, when the back part of the bottom of the foot (the heel) contacts the ground.

Hypoglycemia - low sugar levels in the blood.

Hyperthyroidism - overactivity of the thyroid gland.

Iliac - referring to the ilium, the wing like portion of the hipbone (the flank).

Infections - the presence and growth of abnormal numbers of bacteria, viruses or parasites within the body. Classic signs are pain, redness, heat, swelling and impaired function. Excessive growth of the organisms involved leads to a disruption of the body's defensive mechanisms and lowered resistance.

Initial Swing - the first subphase of the swing phase of gait. It occurs at the beginning of the swing phase, when you have acceleration of movement as the foot clears the ground and the leg moves forward.

Insoles in a shoe, the foot bed or surfaces upon which the bottom of the foot rests. Some have good shock-absorbing material under the ball and heel, and usually are removable. Some conform to your foot also. These are also known as sock liners.

Inversion - turning inward of a part of the body towards the midline of the body.

Inverted - a part of the body is turned inward towards the midline of the body.

Joints the place in which two or more connecting bones are joined. The hip, knee, elbow are some examples.

Knock-kneed - also known as genu valgum. When standing, the bones of the legs are bending inward, the knees are touching or very close together and the ankles are apart more than considered normal.

Last - basic form over which a shoe is fabricated. Its shape and characteristics determine how a shoe fits, feels and wears on a foot. Gives a shoe its shape. Modern day lasts are made of plastics.

Ligaments - the tough connective tissue in the body that holds bones together.

Lumbar - the portion of the spine which is in the lower back. There are five vertebrae.

Lumbar Lordosis - excessive arching of the lower back (lumbar) area. This usually results in the abdomen protruding prominently.

M.R.I. - Magnetic Resonance Imaging. A special technique for viewing internal organs using no radioactive rays.

Massage Therapist - a person trained in the various forms of massage for therapeutic purposes, such as restoring power and movement, breaking up adhesions, improving circulation.

Midsole the layer of material, between the outsole and insole of a shoe, to which the upper is usually attached. Provides most of the shock absorption capabilities of the shoe, and also is used to provide stability and motion control.

Midstance - the second part of the stance phase of gait, when the body's weight is moving over the middle (midfoot) of the foot.

Midswing - the second subphase of the swing phase of gait. This occurs when the swing leg is next to the leg on the ground.

Muscle spasm - an abrupt or forceful contraction of a muscle. Can last for minutes to hours and sometimes days. Usually accompanied by varying degrees of pain.

Musculoskeletal System - that system of the body involving the bones, joints, cartilage, muscles, tendons, ligaments and nerves that supply them.

Myositis - inflammation of a muscle.

Naturalist - a non-medical practitioner who claims to be able to cure illness by utilizing natural remedies derived from foods, herbs, light, and water, etc.

Navicular - a boat-shaped bone on the inside of the foot, towards the back.

Neurologist - a physician who specializes in diseases of the nervous system.

Orthopedics - the branch of medicine concerned with diseases and conditions involving muscles, tendons, joints, ligaments, cartilage, bones and the nerves that supply them.

Orthotics - biomechanical orthopedic devices which are used to control and compensate for inefficient foot/leg biomechanical functioning.

Osteopath- a person who practices a branch of healing, that believes the interdependence of the function and structure of the body is essential for good general health and well being. Osteopaths often treat disease by concentrating on the bones, muscles and joints.

Outsole- the bottom of the shoe that comes in contact with the external surfaces on which you are walking or running. It supplies durability and traction qualities to a shoe.

Pain Storm - reoccurrence of symptoms that had receded for a period of time.

Partially - not complete.

Pediatrics - branch of medicine that deals with the growth and development of the child through adolescence. Also encompasses the understanding, diagnosis, treatment and prevention of diseases, injuries and defects of children.

Pelvis - the boney ring formed by the two hip bones and the sacrum and coccyx.

Pelvic Tilt - hip tilt; pronated hands, hands are turned outward.

Periostitis - inflammation of the tissue (periosteum) covering bones.

Physiatrist - a physician who specializes in physical medicine and rehabilitation.

Physical Therapist - a person professionally trained in the utilization of physical agents and exercise for therapeutic and rehabilitative purposes.

Pigeon toed - toeing in; the toes and feet pointed inward or towards each other.

Podiatrist - a health care specialist who diagnoses/treats diseases and musculoskeletal disorders that affect and/or are manifested in a person's feet.

Post - a wedge of material that is applied to the underside of a posture control orthotic to increase the supportive/controlling effect of the device upon the foot and body.

Posterior Chain - muscles in the back of the body.

Posting - applying a wedge of material to the underside of a posture control orthotic, to increase the supportive/controlling effect of the device upon the foot and body.

Postural Collapse - a term used to describe five skeletal system changes that occur in stages, are progressive and may not be obvious in all cases. They are: excessive pronation of the feet, knock-knees, sway back, hunched shoulders and head thrust forward.

Posture Control Orthotics (PCOs) - custom made orthosis form fitted to a person's foot. They are a unique type of orthotic that is a class II mechanical lever designed to increase foot-to-ground contact, thereby decreasing excessive pronation of the foot, and hence, upper body dysfunction. By applying mechanical engineering principles, a specific amount of vertical lift is applied to the bottom of the inside front of the foot through the orthotics.

Posture Control Orthotics Stage Therapy -incremental orthotic changes, where vertical lift is applied to the inside ball of the foot through a Posture Control Orthotic. This is done to increase foot to ground contact.

Posture Control Orthotic Therapy - first incorporates the use of posture control orthotics to stabilize the subtalar joint (the joint below the ankle in the foot), which in turn leads to stability of the pelvic (low back/hip) joint, thereby stabilizing the entire skeletal system. Second, it identifies the other perpetuating factors that can lead to recurrent postural pains/chronic pain syndromes foot to jaw. The end result is a reversal of the negative effects of postural collapse and a change in the biomechanics of the entire body.

Pronated Hands - hands are turned outward.

Pronation- the foot rolls inward and downward as the arch lowers a little. The leg rotates inward and the kneecap turns inward. This allows the foot to become flexible (loose), to absorb shock and adapt to the surface we are walking on.

Propulsion - the third and last part of the stance phase of gait, when the weight is in the front of the foot. This part of the foot propels the body forward to the next step.

Psoriatic Dermatitis - a non-contagious, chronic skin disease, characterized by reddish, silvery patches located on the chest, knees and elbows. It may come and go throughout a person's life.

Rearfoot Varum - the outside of the heel is on the ground and the inside is off the ground a certain amount of degrees or millimeters.

Relaxin - a hormone secreted in the third trimester of pregnancy which causes relaxation of ligaments.

Sacroiliac Joint - the area where the sacrum and the iliac bones form a joint. These areas are on either side of the spine, in the lower back region.

Sacrum - a curved triangular bone composed of five united vertebrae, situated between the last lumbar vertebrae above and the coccyx below and the hip bones on each side. This forms the back of the pelvis.

Sciatica- pain along the sciatic nerve on either side of the body, from the low back down the leg.

Scoliosis - curvature of the spine.

Septic Polyarthritis - the simultaneous inflammation of several joints that are infected.

Shimming - adding a wedge of material to the underside of a posture control orthotic to increase the supportive/controlling effect of the device upon the foot and body.

Spinal Fusion - an operation joining the bones of the spinal column (the vertebrae) together. This makes the spinal column rigid.

Spine - the back bone or spinal column.

Spinal Column - the backbone or spine.

Spondylolisthesis - slipping forward of a vertebra due to a lack of bone.

Spondylolysis - a lack of bone in either the upper or lower part of a vertebra.

Sprain - a tear, rupture or an excessive stretching of a muscle, ligament or joint.

Stance Phase - that part of the gait cycle when the foot is bearing weight and is on the ground. It occurs from heel contact to toe-off (propulsion) of the same foot. It represents about sixty percent of the total gait cycle.

Strain - muscular pain due to excessive stretching or overuse.

Supination - the foot rolls upward and outward. The arch rises a little. The leg rotates outward, and the knee cap turns outward. This allows the foot to become rigid (stable), in order to lift the weight of the body and move it forward.

Sway Back - excessive arching of the back.

Swing Phase - that part of the gait cycle when the foot is off the ground. It occurs from toe-off (end of propulsion) to heel contact of the same foot. It represents forty percent of the total gait cycle.

Talus - the bone on top of the heel bone or calcaneus. Part of the ankle joint; joins the foot to the leg at the ankle.

Temps - temporary elevation added to the inside of a Posture Control Orthotic. It is used to increase the supportive/controlling effect of the device upon the foot and body.

Tendinitis - inflammation of a tendon.

Tendons - the fibrous portion of muscle which attaches the muscle to bone.

Terminal Swing - the third and final subphase of the swing phase of gait. Occurs when you have a slowing down or deceleration of the leg as it is preparing itself to make contact with the supportive surface (the ground).

Thoracic Kyphosis - curvature of the thoracic spine (chest region) in a front to back direction. Also known as humpback.

Thorax - the chest.

Tibial Varum - the lower legs are in a bowlegged position, i.e., the upper parts of the lower legs are farther apart than they should be. The lower parts are too close together.

Transmandibular Joint Dysfunction (TMJ) - improper functioning of the jaw joint.

Transparency - cannot detect (feel) when Posture Control Orthotics are in one's shoes.

Trigger Points - an area of irritation, usually within a skeletal muscle; when pressed and/or squeezed, is very tender itself and often causes referred pain to another area.

Triple Arthrodesis - surgical fusion of three major joints in the foot just below the ankle. These are the talonavicular, calcaneal-cuboid and the talocalcaneal.

Tumor - an abnormal growth or mass resulting from an excessive multiplication of cells.

Uric Acid - a normal chemical constituent of the blood. When present in excessive amounts, it may be associated with gout.

Vertebra - one of the bones forming the spinal column in the back.

Vertebrae - bones forming the spinal column. Plural of Vertebra.

Vertebral - of or pertaining to the vertebra or vertebrae.

Vertical Height - the straight up, topmost point of something.

Vertical Lift - material that adds height to the underside of a Posture Control Orthotic to increase the supportive/controlling effect of the device upon the foot and body.

Walking - also referred to as gait. Repetitive acts of one's body falling forward, foot contacting the ground, and catching ourselves. In the meantime, the opposite foot and leg are moving off the ground.

Wedge - material that is applied to the underside of a Posture Control Orthotic to increase the supportive/controlling effect of the device upon the foot and body.

Bibliography

Anderson, B. *Stretching.* Fullerton, CA. 1975.

Anderson, J. E. *Grant's Atlas Of Anatomy.* 7th ed. Baltimore, MD: Williams & Wilkins, 1978.

Birnbaum, J. S. *The Musculoskeletal Manual.* New York: Academic Press, 1982.

Bottle, R. R. "An Interpretation Of The Pronation Syndrome And Foot Types Of Patients With Low Back Pain." *JAMPA* 71 (1981): 243-253.

Brody, D. M. "Running Injuries." *Ciba Clinical Symposia* Vol 32 (4) (1980).

Cyriax, J. *Text Book of Orthopedic Medicine - Volume 1.* East Sussex, England: Bailliere Tindell, 1978.

Dannenberg, H. J. "Temporomandibular Joint (TMJ) Dysfunction Syndrome as a Result of Gait Malfunction: A Case Study." *Current Podiatric Medicine,* July 1988.

Delacerda, F. G., and O. D. Wikoff. "Effect Of Lower Extremity Asymmetry On The Kinematics Of Gait." *J Orthop Sports Pys Ther* 3 (1982): 105-107.

Green, C. S. "Myofascial Pain-Dysfunction Syndrome: The Evolution of Concepts." *The Temporomandibular Joint.* Ed. B. G. Sarnat and D. M. Laskin. Springfield, IL: Charles C. Thomas. 1980. Chapter 13.

Greenawalt, Monte H. *Spinal Pelvic Stabilization.* Copyright 1987 by Foot Levelers, Inc.

Hiemeyer K., Lutz, R., and H. Menninger. "Dependence Of Tender Points Upon Posture — Key To The Understanding Of Fibromyalgia Syndrome." *J Man Med* 5 (1990):169-174.

Hoppenfield, S. *Physical Examination Of The Spine and Extremities.* New York: Appleton-Century-Crofts. 1976.

LeVeau et al. *Biomechanics of Human Motion.* Philadelphia: Saunders. 1977.

Magee, D. J. *Orthopedic Physical Assessment.* Philadelphia: W. B. Saunders Co. 1987.

Merck & Co., Inc. *The Merck Manual of Diagnosis and Therapy.* Editor-in-chief Robert Berkow, M.D. Rahway, NJ: Merck Research Laboratories. 1992.

Peterson, J. A. and J. Wheeler. *The Goodbye Back Pain Handbook.* Grand Rapids, MI: Masters Press. 1988.

Prevention Magazine Editorial Staff. *Symptoms: Their Causes And Cures.* Emmaus, PA: Rodale Press, Inc. 1994.

Root, L. and T. Kiernam. *Oh, My Aching Back.* New York: NAL Penguin Inc. 1973.

Ross, T. and W. A. Rossi. *Professional Shoe Fitting.* New York: National Shoe Retailers Association. 1984.

Rothbart, B. "Biomechanical Medicine: Its Application In Chronic Pain Patients." *BioMedicine,* Vol. 1, Winter 1993.

Rothbart, B. and K. Yerrat. "An Innovative Mechanical Approach To Treating Chronic Knee Pain: A BioImplosion Model." *AJPM,* Vol. 4 No. 3. (July 1994): 123-128

Sarrafian, S. K. *Anatomy Of The Foot And Ankle.* Philadelphia: J. B. Lippincott Co. 1983.

Schneider, M. J. and M. D. Sussman. *The Athlete's Health Care Book - From the Hip Down.* Washington, DC: Acropolis Books Ltd. 1983.

Sgarlato, T. E. *A Compendium Of Podiatric Biomechanics.* San Francisco: California College of Podiatric Medicine. March 1971.

Taylor, P. M. and D. K. Taylor. *Conquering Athletic Injuries.* Champaign, IL: Leisure Press. 1988.

Thurston & Harris. "Normal Kinematics Of The Lumbar Spine And Pelvic Spine." *Spine.* June 1983.

Timm, R. "BioImplosion And Postural Control." *BioMedicine,* Vol. 1. Winter 1993.

Travell, J. G. and D. G. Simmons. "Myofascial Pain And Dysfunction." *The Trigger Point Manual* Volumes 1 & 2. Copyright 1992.

Index

Neck pains, 30, 123
Neuroma, 25

Orthopedic supports, 118
Osgood-Schlatter's disease, 28
Osteodegenerative arthritis, 31
Outsole, 87
Overuse
    sports injuries, 32
    syndrome, 106

Pain storm, 36
Pelvis, 14-15
Physical therapy, 115-118
Pigeon-toed, 79
Posting, 35
Posts, 37
Postural collapse, 18-20, 22, 80
Posture
    control orthotics, 34-41
    reading, 94
    sex, 97
    sitting, 93-94, 98
    sleeping, 95-96
    standing, 91-92
    traveling, 95
Posture control orthotic therapy
    contraindications, 37-38
    definition, 34-36, 38-39
Posture control orthotic stage
    therapy, 35
Pregnancy and postural pains, 111-112
Pronation
    definition, 11-14
    excessive, 16, 18-19, 22, 81
Propulsion, 12-13
Psychological factors, 113-114
Pubic bone, 15

Referred pain, 32
R.I.C.E., 118

Sacroiliac joint, 19
Sacrum, 15
Sciatica, 29
Scoliosis, 29

Sesamoiditis, 25
Shimming, 35
Shin splints, 27
Shoes
    fitting process, 82-83
    high-heel, 85-86, 99
    old, 84
    posture control orthotics, 86
    specific types of, 85
Shoulder pains, 30
Spine, 14
Spondylolisthesis, 29
Stance phase, 12
Stress fracture
    femur, 28
    foot, 26
    leg, 27
    thigh, 28
Stretching, 109-110
Subtalar joint, 11
Supination, 11, 13-14
Swing
    leg, 14
    phase, 12, 14

Talus, 18
Target heart rate, 103
Temps, 37
Tendinitis, 27-18
Tensor fascia latae - iliotibial band
    syndrome, 28
Terminal swing, 14
Thigh injuries, 28
Thoracic
    kyphosis, 20
    outlet syndrome, 29
Thorax, 15
Toe-off, 13
Transmandibular joint dysfunction
    (TMJ), 30

Upper body, 16

Vertical lift, 35, 37, 39

Walking, 10, 11, 15
Wedging, 37
Whiplash, 30